Ethics and Evidence-Based Medicine

"At its core, evidence-based practice rests on a supposition which, while probably true, itself has unclear evidentiary support."

A quarter-century of outcomes research, systematic reviews, and research synthesis have reshaped medicine and other health professions, even as they have been subjected to vigorous and vehement criticism. The growth of evidence-based medicine has occurred against a backdrop of health care reform, managed care, cost containment, and quality improvement, and clinicians have been urged to adopt the rigors of science while remaining true to their "clinical judgment." This tension – between efforts to make medical practice more scientific and the suspicions of many clinicians – has caused one of the greatest practical and ethical challenges in the history of the health professions. This incisive book reviews the history and conceptual origins of evidence-based practice and discusses key ethical issues that arise in clinical practice, public health, and health policy.

Essential reading for all physicians, and practitioners in epidemiology and public health, it will also be suitable as a text in medical and public health school courses on evidence-based practice.

Kenneth W. Goodman is founder and director of the University of Miami's Bioethics Program and its Pan-American Bioethics Initiative. He is also co-director of the University's Program in Business, Government and Professional Ethics, and holds appointments in the Departments of Medicine, Philosophy, Epidemiology and Public Health, and the School of Nursing. He is editor of *Ethics, Computing and Medicine* (Cambridge, 1998), and the author of articles on bioethics, the philosophy of science and computing.

Ethics and
Evidence-Based Medicine

Fallibility and Responsibility in
Clinical Science

Kenneth W. Goodman

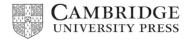

PUBLISHED BY THE PRESS SYNDICATE OF THE UNIVERSITY OF CAMBRIDGE
The Pitt Building, Trumpington Street, Cambridge, United Kingdom

CAMBRIDGE UNIVERSITY PRESS
The Edinburgh Building, Cambridge CB2 2RU, UK
40 West 20th Street, New York, NY 10011–4211, USA
477 Williamstown Road, Port Melbourne, VIC 3207, Australia
Ruiz de Alarcón 13, 28014 Madrid, Spain
Dock House, The Waterfront, Cape Town 8001, South Africa

http://www.cambridge.org

First published 2003

Printed in the United Kingdom at the University Press, Cambridge

Typeface Minion 10.5/13 pt   *System* QuarkXPress™ [SE]

A catalogue record for this book is available from the British Library

Library of Congress Cataloguing in Publication data

Goodman, Kenneth W., 1954–
Ethics and evidence-based medicine : fallibility and responsibility in clinical science /
Kenneth W. Goodman.
    p. cm.
Includes bibliographical references and index.
ISBN 0 521 81933 4 (hbk.) – ISBN 0 521 79653 9 (pbk.)
1. Medical ethics. 2. Evidence-based medicine. I. Title.

R725.5 G66 2002
174′.2–dc21   2002067402

ISBN 0 521 81933 4 hardback
ISBN 0 521 79653 9 paperback

Every effort has been made in preparing this book to provide accurate and up-to-date
information that is in accord with accepted standards and practice at the time of
publication. Nevertheless, the authors, editors and publisher can make no warranties that
the information contained herein is totally free from error, not least because clinical
standards are constantly changing through research and regulation. The authors, editors
and publisher therefore disclaim all liability for direct or consequential damages resulting
from the use of material contained in this book. Readers are strongly advised to pay
careful attention to information provided by the manufacturer of any drugs or equipment
that they plan to use.

For Allison and Jacqueline
Evidence of so much that is worth believing

in the service of human health care raises ethical issues. Largest among these is that scientific uncertainty itself presents clinicians with ethical challenges and issues. This is less important when there is plenty of evidentiary warrant for clinical decisions, but at other times, it seems, we can live and die by the slenderest of epistemological threads. With very few exceptions, these issues have not been addressed in the literatures of either medicine or ethics.

The book has this structure:

After a survey of the origins of evidence-based practice (Beddoes in the eighteenth century, Louis in the nineteenth, and Cochrane in the twentieth), Chapter 1 makes a case for linking clinical and scientific knowledge on the one hand, and morality on the other; it is the core theme of the book. Along the way, we touch on some of the roles of, and relations among, information, evidence, expertise, specialization, progress, communication, and error. The project is not as grand as that might suggest, however, and the conclusion is actually quite straightforward, if not simple: Ignorance can be blameworthy.

That said, *reducing* ignorance is not such a simple affair. Contemporary biomedical science – including the means of reporting results, the social and professional engines that drive scientific publication, and the tools for pulling it all together – is a great and complicated affair. Chapter 2 tries to make some sense of it, and of the research synthesis revolution that has transformed the medical sciences over the past quarter-century. Such a revolution, with its systematic reviews and meta-analyses, has the goal of providing better or stronger warrant for clinical beliefs. Like other revolutions, however, partisans on all sides have an interest in making matters seem simpler than they really are.

Chapter 3 examines in greater detail the exciting and vexing problem of "evidence about evidence" (called "meta-evidence" here). From the quality of initial research and peer review to the edifices built by combining, concatenating, and otherwise melding sometimes disparate inquiries, we are faced with a practical and conceptual problem of the greatest magnitude. One solution to the problem requires that ordinary clinicians get a handle on the debates that consume investigators and scholars, if for no other reason than to have (at least the beginning of) an answer to the question, "*What kind of scientific evidence is a meta-analysis or a systematic review, and how best should these tools be incorporated in research and clinical practice?*"

A traditional picture of clinical investigation or human subjects research has folk in white coats moving between hospital bed and laboratory. But

Preface

It is surely one of the best – one of the most interesting and most important – questions in the history of human inquiry. It can be asked as plainly as we like, yet be disputed as fiercely as any, ever:

Why do you believe what you do, and not something else?

We can ask this question generally or specifically, grandly or trivially. It can, for instance, be about the origin of the universe or the fate of next season's marigolds, the existence of God or the prospects for the Miami Hurricanes or the Tottenham Hotspurs, the best treatment for breast cancer or the worst way to play bridge. The question is sometimes a request for reasons or evidence or, sometimes, both (raising the further questions as to whether and when a bit of evidence *is* a reason . . .).

Like most good questions, the fact that it is simple to ask does not mean that it is easy to answer. This is a pity, because when we are talking about life and health and death, and not marigolds, football, or bridge, then it would have been nice if the answer were simple.

Nevertheless, and simple or not, clinicians have a bold-faced duty to answer it. The day is gone when a physician or nurse might justify a clinical decision by offering as reason (or purported reason) a story that begins in any of the following ways:

It seems to me . . .
In my experience . . .
I was taught . . .

There are a number of reasons for this change in the evidentiary standards of clinical practice. First, there is just a lot more evidence than there used to be. Second, the evidence is better than it once was. Last, it is easier to get one's hands on this evidence than in the pre-Internet days of yore. There may be other reasons. In aggregate, they point to the thesis that motivates this book, namely that the deployment or application of scientific evidence

Contents

information technology is changing research as it is changing all other aspects of contemporary life. Chapter 4 reviews some of these changes and attempts to locate them against the background we have grown familiar with, i.e., uncertainty, causation, and error avoidance. This chapter deals with issues including recruitment of subjects on the World Wide Web, data mining, bioinformatics (or the use of computers in genetics research and practice), and, in a field we call "emergency public health informatics," early warning systems for bioterror attacks.

Science and practice are often about discovering, recognizing, and following patterns. The growth of evidence-based practice and its new evidence has, however, engendered an opposition movement and a countervailing "new skepticism" that seeks to impeach the requirements embodied in practice guidelines and other clinical pattern-following rules. Chapter 5 has the task of making clear that the hoary confusion regarding the extent to which medicine is an art or a science is a relic of murkier times and not a useful way to think about the management of uncertainty in clinical practice. Debates over practice guidelines, especially in managed care and the law, must move beyond simple advocacy by proponents and equally facile skepticism by detractors. Evidence-based practice emerges as "an earnest and honest attempt to help clinicians do best, what they already were committed to doing well."

Chapter 6 connects the debates over evidence-based practice to issues in public policy. We use three case studies, which involve research on environmental tobacco smoke, screening mammography, and otitis media – cases chosen because of their difficulty and the controversy surrounding them. This chapter attempts to anticipate future human subjects research, especially drug discovery and genomics, in light of the needs of population-based research and the implications of such research for public policy. The by-now familiar challenge of clinical uncertainty is applied to communities and health policy.

The duties of clinicians, investigators, research synthesizers, and review boards are linked in many and various ways. Chapter 7 takes our understanding of evidence and fallibility and concludes that, as a practical matter, each of these groups does its duty when it maximizes quality, minimizes bias, and manages uncertainty. Society, too, has a duty – to provide for more and better research, as well as the means to make better sense of systematic science.

Kenneth W. Goodman
University of Miami

Acknowledgments

I am grateful to a number of individuals and institutions. Foremost thanks are due to Norman Altman at the University of Miami for helping to make possible the environment in which such a project could be undertaken. Alex Jadad at the University of Toronto, a wise and creative thinker regarding the role of evidence in health care, has been generous with advice and encouragement. Richard Barling of Cambridge University Press has also been a source of encouragement and, fortunately, patience. Gary Dunbar's assistance was invaluable in many ways, not least in tracking down and sorting out a variety of online and other resources (not everything is on the Web, thank goodness). Sarah Dunstall lent a sharp eye and gentle ear to the manuscript.

Ideas from parts of this book were tried out in tutorials for the American Medical Informatics Association, in grand rounds in pediatrics departments at the University of Miami and the State University of New York at Buffalo, and at the annual PriMed Conference sponsored by the University of Miami and Harvard University. Finally, some of the work represented in Chapter 4 was supported by the US Department of Veterans Affairs under its state-of-the-art research program; other aspects of work in that chapter were supported by a National Institutes of Health grant (T15 AI07591).

Foundations and history of evidence-based practice

It isn't what we don't know that gives us trouble, it's what we know that ain't so.

Will Rogers

This chapter will locate systematic science and evidence-based medicine against the background of biomedical research in the second half of the twentieth century. The growth of this research paralleled and in some ways forced the evolution of current standards for communicating the results of scientific inquiry (i.e., the emergence of peer review and the expansion of the number of research programs, journals, books, etc.). The research raises interesting issues about the role and nature of expertise and medical knowledge, and it has led to a vast tableau of practice guidelines, critical pathways, consensus statements, and assorted other scientifically based imperatives for the care of individual patients. These imperatives are increasingly linked to physician and institution reimbursement. Where the stakes are highest, as in clinical medicine and public health, these forces assume special importance for ethics and public policy.

Before it became a movement, or a cause, evidence-based medicine (EBM) was a kind of cognitive itch: a troublesome doubt that follows from the realizations that humans are fallible, that scientific knowledge increases and that medical decisions sometimes have very high stakes. If you make a mistake, your patient might die. Less ominous, even if they do not die, patients are often paying for physicians' services, either through taxes or by putting cash on the barrel in one way or another. Failure to know what one is doing then becomes a kind of rip-off or scam. These realizations tend to focus the attention of most clinicians.

Patients die or otherwise come to grief all the time, of course. A bad or unhappy outcome can be the result of any of a large ensemble of causes:
• Ignorance, carelessness or inattention (individual)
• Ignorance, carelessness or inattention (collective)
• Futility
• Incompetence

- Conflict of interest
- Deception (by a patient)
- Malign intent

There may be others, but we are concerned in any case with the first two. (Note that the first two are cognate with the increasingly important work on medical *error* or mistakes, in which various forms of inattention and failures of institutional process are identified as responsible for mistakes and consequent harms (see Bosk 1981, the locus classicus; and Kohn, Corrigan, and Donaldson 2000). We shall return to error at the end of the chapter.)

To have evidence is to have some conceptual warrant for a belief or action. This says nothing so far about the *quality* of the evidence and hence the strength of the warrant. To be in a state of ignorance is to have false beliefs or to lack beliefs one way or another about the way the world works. If I do not have the belief that germs cause disease, and if germs do cause disease, then I am ignorant of the fact that germs cause disease. Now, this would be a grave shortcoming in a twenty-first century physician, but not in one practicing in the fourth century BC, say. This is because my twenty-first century ignorance is individual and my fourth century ignorance is collective. Twenty-five centuries ago no-one knew that germs cause disease; now, everyone (at least everyone who is practicing medicine) does, or should.

At any rate, the demand that clinicians know what they are doing, more or less, is an ancient one and it has, from the beginning, been couched as a *moral* imperative. The Hippocratic Oath (likely *not* written by Hippocrates) may be read as a celebration of teachers and education at least as much as an itemization of duties and virtues. When the oath-taker vows to "regard him who has taught me this technē as equal to my parents," she is celebrating the transmission of knowledge; when she promises not to "cut, and certainly not those suffering from stone, but I will cede [this] to men [who are] practitioners of this activity," it is a vow not to practice beyond one's knowledge or capacity (translation by Von Staden 1996).

The Oath of Maimonides, after the twelfth century physician, rabbi, and philosopher Moses Maimonides, entreats, "Grant me the strength, time and opportunity always to correct what I have acquired, always to extend its domain; for knowledge is immense and the spirit of man can extend indefinitely to enrich itself daily with new requirements" (translation by Friedenwald 1917). Surely this should be read as a plea not to fall too far behind in monitoring the shifting landscape of medical evidence, a medieval anticipation of the importance – the *moral* importance – of continuing medical education.

It could not be otherwise. The intersection of knowledge and health points to a moral imperative because idiosyncratic ignorance causes or allows people to be harmed. An individual clinician's ignorance becomes blameworthy in part because his or her patients would have fared better elsewhere, in the hands of another whose greater knowledge (or lesser ignorance) would have saved the day. Now, this raises interesting questions about how far behind one might lapse without blame, and we will return to them later. The notion is important to us now because we want to distinguish idiosyncratic ignorance from community or collective ignorance.

What physicians don't know[1]

At its core, evidence-based practice rests on a supposition which, while probably true, itself has unclear evidentiary support.

The demand that clinicians make the most of evidence – or even high-quality scientific evidence – in patient care is a demand that catches our attention only if it can be shown that they were not doing so already. One might try a little experiment with a friend or family member whose work is wholly outside health care . . . mention that evidence-based medicine has become a profession-wide movement to try to get doctors to practice in accord with, well, the evidence. The hypothesis is that you will be met by confusion if not outright incomprehension: "What were they basing their decisions on before all this?" Well, what indeed? In fact, of course, the healing professions have always, albeit in one degree or another, been based on evidence. It is just that there has been precious little of it, and it hasn't been any good. In some (but not all) cases, it has been just enough to distinguish physicians from shamans.

Thomas Beddoes and Pierre Louis

The likely true but undersupported supposition at the core of evidence-based medicine is that most health care is (or, until comparatively recently, was) not evidence based. This means either of two things: (1) There is no (adequate) evidence available to support clinical inferences, or there is, somewhere, but clinicians have no access to it; (2) the truth may be out there, but it doesn't matter if we cannot lay our hands on it. The latter is among the targets of post-Enlightenment medical epistemology and a celebration of human experience and open communication. We can probably trace the intellectual birth of evidence-based practice to Thomas Beddoes (1760–1808), the English physician known in part for his "Pneumatic Institution" for the study of the medical use of gases[2] and, perhaps more importantly, for his criticism of turn-of-the-century medical practice.

Beddoes argued that eighteenth century medicine had become hidebound, stagnant, and secretive (Porter 1992). Here is how the medical historian Roy Porter summarizes the points Beddoes makes in his 1808 "Letter to the Right Honourable Sir Joseph Banks . . . on the Causes and Removal of the Prevailing Discontents, Imperfections, and Abuses, in Medicine":

Beddoes proposed two solutions. First, systematic collection and indexing of medical facts. "Why should not reports be transmitted at fixed periods from all the hospitals and medical charities in the kingdom to a central board?" Other "charitable establishments for the relief of the indigent sick" must also supply information, as should physicians at large. Data should be processed by a paid clerical staff, and made freely available. Seminars should be held. The stimulus to comparison and criticisms would sift good practice from bad. "What would be the effect", Beddoes mused, of "register offices, not exactly for receiving votive tablets, like certain ancient temples, but in which attestations, both of the good and of the evil, that appears to be done by practitioners of medicine, should be deposited?" Without effective information storage, retrieval and dissemination, medicine would never take its place amongst the progressive sciences. "To lose a single fact may be to lose many lives. Yet ten thousand, perhaps, are lost for one that is preserved; and all for want of a system among our theatres of disease, combined with the establishment of a national bank of medical wealth, where each individual practitioner may deposit his grains of knowledge, and draw out, in return, the stock, accumulated by all his brethren.". . . Second, to complement his medical bank, Beddoes urged his fellows to publish more . . . . (Porter 1992: 10, notes omitted)

Data sharing . . . collecting and archiving . . . analysis and reporting . . . publishing . . . It seems that the good Dr. Beddoes was calling for a comprehensive system of medical information management. Moreover, he was calling for such a system because he believed, with good warrant, that the medical science of his day was shortchanging – was harming – patients, and that it could be better. Information becomes evidence when it applies to, bears on, or constitutes a reason for (dis)believing the truth of a proposition. If we are talking about propositions related to life, death, pain, disability, and so forth, then it is just a few short steps until we identify a *duty* to collect and share information that bears on those propositions.

Thomas Beddoes is suggesting a moral link between information management and medical practice. He is proposing outcomes research and fantasizing about systematic reviews; demanding databases and hoping for data mining; insisting on broader dissemination, and doing so two centuries ago, or before the World Wide Web would, at least in principle, put every publication on every desktop.

Somewhat after Beddoes, in 1834, Pierre Charles Alexandre Louis (1787–1872), published his *Essay on Clinical Instruction*. The foundation of what was for a while called the "Numerical Method," it, along with his other works, also constituted a cornerstone in the history of clinical evaluation. Louis apparently performed the first chart reviews ("outcomes research" if you like) and thereby produced evidence to undermine beliefs about bloodletting, not least the notion that bleeding cured cholera[3] (Porter 1996; Weatherall 1996):

> As to different methods of treatment, it is possible for us to assure ourselves of the superiority of one or other . . . by enquiring if the greater number of individuals have been cured by one means than another. Here it is necessary to count. And it is, in great part at least, because hitherto this method has not at all, or rarely been employed, that the science of therapeutics is so uncertain. (Louis 1834: 26–28)

It is simple arithmetic, but it is systematic enough to be credited as an intellectual parent by Osler (1985 [1897]) and as a key antecedent of evidence-based practice in a major text and exposition (Sackett et al. 2000). Indeed, it might be possible to blame Osler for contributing to, if not originating, the belief that the acquisition of evidence is a simple matter:

> Louis introduced what is known as the Numerical Method, a plan which we use every day, though the phrase is not now very often on our lips. The guiding motto of his life was "Ars medica tota in observationibus", in carefully observing facts, carefully collating them, carefully analysing them. To get an accurate knowledge of any disease it is necessary to study a large series of cases and to go into all the particulars – the conditions under which it is met, the subjects specially liable, the various symptoms, the pathological changes, the effects of drugs. This method, so simple, so self-evident, we owe largely to Louis. (Osler 1985 [1897]: 193)

We see at any rate the several forces at work as medical science moved from innocence to awareness of the varied and gorgeously useful data to be teased from clinical experience.

From Beddoes and Louis to Cochrane

What followed, albeit as a result of a number of forces disconnected from Beddoes and his dicta and Louis and his data, was an industry that published the cases and observations of clinicians, often in journals linked to professional societies (Bynum and Wilson 1992). Still, it took until the middle of the twentieth century before medical science was to evolve the tool we call the randomized clinical trial and which we tend to regard as the gold standard for generating the information which we then turn into evidence (British Medical Journal 1998).[4] But what had failed to evolve was a system for making the information-evidence alchemy reliable and broadly available. The failure was frank and unavoidable: Clinicians needed help in muddling through the vast and often contradictory mess of information that might or might not drift across the transom.

What has emerged over the past quarter-century is a series of pronouncements about the percentage of health care that is based on (high-quality or even gold standard) evidence. This percentage is always very low – it ranges from 10% to 25% of medical decisions. The numbers leave us slack-jawed. If clinicians' decisions are based on (high-quality) evidence only 10% or 25% or even 50% of the time, then what on earth is guiding the rest of the decisions in which pain, suffering, disability, and life hang in the balance?

The numbers matter, because if they are wrong we have less to worry about, and if they are right we had better get moving.

The origin of the numbers is obscure. At a delightful and illuminating UK-based website, "What proportion of healthcare is evidence based?", the question elicits pointers to a broad variety of sources that try to establish the percentage with some degree of, well, evidence. The origin of the minimal-evidence claim is worth savoring:

"The 10–25% of medical decisions are evidence-based" comes from a series of conjectures, many of them humorous, starting back in the 70's. For example, in an exchange between giants of epidemiology, Kerr White . . . and Archie Cochrane . . . in Wellington, NZ, Kerr had just suggested that "only about 15–20% of physicians' interventions were supported by objective evidence that they did more good than harm" when Archie interrupted him with: "Kerr, you're a damned liar! [Y]ou know it isn't more than 10%." (Booth et al. 1999)

Other sources of the claim include the US Office of Technology Assessment (10–20%; Office of Technology Assessment 1978) and the Institute of

Medicine (2–25% varying by strength of evidence and consensus; Field and Lohr 1992). But we might as well trace the contemporary unease, the epistemological gap, the cognitive itch to Archie Cochrane's observation and complaint: "It is surely a great criticism of our profession that we have not organised a critical summary, by specialty or subspecialty, adapted periodically, of all relevant randomized controlled trials" (Cochrane 1979; cf. Cochrane 1972). There is a sense in which Cochrane, born in Galashiels, Scotland, in 1909, a century after Beddoes' death, has done as much as any other individual to reshape health education and practice. Since his death in 1988, his core idea has mutated from insight to tribute to movement to professional imperative.

Such a simple idea, so straightforwardly expressed, so intuitively compelling: It was a great criticism indeed that there were, two millennia after the physicians at Kos, few collective accounts or reports that what clinicians did had any demonstrable scientific traction. It is surely one of the great oversights in the history of human inquiry and applied epistemology. Indeed, even Beddoes' proposed system for rudimentary data collection and outcomes research had not been instituted in some quarters, two centuries later.

To be sure, the fact that a claim or practice is not supported by (adequate) evidence does not mean that it is false. But it does mean that practitioners have inadequate grounds for believing it to be true or effective. Put differently: The remaining 90% or 75% or whatever percentage of health care that is said not to be evidence based is not necessarily false – only that clinicians lack (adequate) justification to assert it to be true and perhaps to practice as if they knew it to be.

Efforts to warrant such assertions have, in less than 25 years, shaped everything from medical reimbursement to resource allocation to managed care to public health to individual decisions by individual clinicians – faced and challenged by vast amounts of health research and by partisan claims about how to make sense of it all.

Observe that Cochrane's complaint here is not that most individual clinicians' beliefs are not supported by evidence. It is that, for all they know, they are! It is therefore a much broader challenge: If the beliefs of clinicians can be linked to evidence, then those links need to be accessible – in an "organized, critical summary." In this sense, Archie Cochrane was not asking for more research or more evidence; he was merely observing that the evidence we already have is removed or disconnected from the people who ought to be using it to take care of sick people.

In terms of the two kinds of ignorance we included in our earlier list of causes of bad outcomes, Cochrane is therefore talking about the first, or individual ignorance (call it "I-I"; collective ignorance will be "C-I"). Now, I-I must, if it is to make any sense, mean something like this:

A clinician is *individually ignorant* of evidence that would affect her practice if she were aware of it, if:
- such evidence has already been acquired by someone, somewhere; and
- the evidence is not secret, and has not been hidden or unpublished/unshared.

We want these two conditions to apply in order to insulate us from cases (as suggested in Chapter 2) in which, say, a discovery had been made but unreported – ignorance of such a discovery would be ignorance that (almost) everyone has and so would be no different in salient respects from collective ignorance:

A clinician is *collectively ignorant* of evidence that would affect her practice if she were aware of it, if:
- such evidence has not been acquired by anyone yet, where "acquired" may include evidence requiring either primary research or knowledge discovery as is attributed to database research, meta-analysis, etc.

In other words, the set or class of people who are collectively ignorant comprises members none of whom has evidence that would affect practice decisions if the evidence were known. Ignorance, like misery, loves company.

There are several ways in which our simple distinction does not cover all eventualities. For instance, in trying to distinguish between having and not-having some evidence, we have adopted a vague and imprecise picture of evidence. It makes no mention of the quality of the evidence, for instance. When we say "evidence that would affect her practice if she were aware of it," we have said nothing about whether our clinician *should* alter her practice in light of it, whether it would be *rational* to do so, etc. These are important questions and we will return to them in Chapter 2. For now, it is adequate to point out that the historical thrust of evidence-based practice owes much to men who were asking for something very basic and obvious.

That something is basic or obvious, however, does not always make it easy to believe.

Health science and the growth of knowledge – the role of "experts"

Even as scientific progress entails scientific change, the reverse is not the case. Some changes are trivial, off the mark, or even destructive or regressive. Evaluating candidates for, and changes in, scientific corpora requires a broad cluster of attributes, most especially knowledge of the science in which an inquiry is conducted and in which the progress is alleged. The conflicting forces of specialized knowledge and interdisciplinary knowledge create a vast cluster of problems for those who would assess scientific change and progress. Such an assessment is precisely what evidence-based medicine demands.

On one obvious reading, the evolution of specialization in medicine has been driven by the great and rapid accumulation of information about the human organism. The effects of this accumulation force us to abandon the hope that individuals might become complete masters of particular disciplines:

In every subject of scientific study the progress of investigation and the accumulation of knowledge must reach a point where it becomes a serious task to master all its facts, or to be acquainted with all that has been written about it. When a great number of zealous observers are bending their energies in a common pursuit, it happens after a time that not the oldest and most eminent among them can possibly attain to a perfect acquaintance with all that is known about it. (Noyes 1865: 59)[5]

In the century-and-a-third since Dr. Noyes reflected thus on the heavy weight of information that increasingly attaches to the good fortune of knowledge, the situation has become somewhat more complicated. Not only has medicine progressed, it has found itself closely allied with disciplines not then imagined. All the while and as ever, going back to Plato and Aristotle, the questions of how to assess medical and other scientific claims, and of who is most fit to communicate the claims, have tended to turn to experts.[6] Now, this could be a problem because it is probably too much to require that ordinary clinicians become experts. If evidence-based practice required this, it would be doomed to failure. It is a more democratic enterprise, requiring that all clinicians take responsibility for their own epistemic warrants. In other contexts, we would call this "education."

Fortunately, there are a number of ways to defang calls to expertise. One is to make the case that "expertise" is akin to "narrowness" or "rigidity."

Another is to undermine the very idea that there is such a thing as expertise, or that it is needed for the purpose at hand.

For instance, regarding the former, the philosopher Paul Feyerabend has condemned experts "who quite naturally confound knowledge with mental rigor mortis" (Feyerabend 1975: 182; cf. Feyerabend 1978). Feyerabend is also reading "authority" for "expert" and this bit of economy links social position with (narrow) epistemological status: better to plague both houses.

Can we successfully set aside the very concept of "expert?" Or, better, does evidence-based medicine even need any expertise?[7] Since a large part of the evidence-based engine requires the synthesis and communication of information by ordinary clinicians, we should look a little more closely at this process of evaluation.

Evaluating progress in medicine

Evidence of progress in medicine and nursing is in some respects less controversial than evidence of progress in physics, genetics, astronomy, psychology, and other sciences. Where quarks, genes, black holes, superegos, and other entities have raised, and continue to raise, difficult problems for those who postulate their existence, structure, and function, the entities of modern medicine lend themselves somewhat less readily to philosophical scavenging. This is emphatically not to argue that medicine offers no or even only few special difficulties for the analysis of new evidence – indeed, as we will see later, scientific uncertainty poses the greatest ethical challenge to evidence-based practice – it is merely to suggest that these difficulties are in some respects harder to come by or more tractable than issues in other sciences. The observation has this to recommend it: To the extent that medicine reduces to chemistry and physics, its deepest problems will not be uniquely medical at all but rather chemical, physical, and so forth.

Still, there are fundamental difficulties in the task under analysis, namely assessing and communicating facts and allegations of progress. No matter how we join the old philosophical debate over progress in science, the question of whether there has been any of it in a given domain will be answered only or best by those who have some set of skills and/or some amount of knowledge.

Consider provisionally that an assessment of progress in a science will require knowledge of the (at least short-term) history of the science and of the events alleged to be progressive. For now, call a person with that knowledge an "expert."

Now suppose there are two kinds of progress – technological and theoretical. Technological progress might be found in the invention of a surgical tool or a drug, even perhaps in the identification of a disease. Theoretical progress will be the acquisition of explanatory knowledge about the structure and function of organs, diseases, systems, and so on. Thus the ancient discovery *that* certain substances had antiseptic properties was an instance of the former; work by Pasteur and Lister increased our understanding of *why* some substances are antiseptic, and so was progressive at the deeper, theoretical level.

We seem therefore to require two different kinds of expert. One teases phenomena from the world, the other learns its secrets. Of course, both of these oversimplified attributes might be found in a single person, as for example in William Harvey, who embodied experimental insights as well as explanatory and theoretical genius. Likewise, if we are lucky, the phenomenon comes to us kit-and-caboodle *with* its explanation and we get both kinds of progress at once. The world is rarely so accommodating, however. (Many errors in the history of science – geocentrism, phlogiston, and the theory of bodily humors come to mind – result from attempts to link too quickly initial phenomena, which might not be genuine, to theories and posits, which enjoy inadequate support. They might be unavoidable.)

The evaluation of medical progress is then a two-fold affair: It is the evaluation of technological progress and theoretical progress. Because every claim or report of a scientific advance ought not to be taken at face value (any individual claim might be wrong), we require some way to judge the truth content and importance of scientific claims. Viewed as a meta-scientific job description, this requirement underlies the work done by journal referees and editors, journalists (popular and specialized), grant administrators, department heads, government officials, and others who must gauge the activity and claims of scientists. Do we need experts for these tasks? In the other direction: Are those who perform these tasks experts?

There are few concepts that are so frequently used and appealed to, and yet so poorly understood, as expertise. This is too bad, because it assumes something we have yet to learn, namely, what it is to be an expert, that is, what constitutes expertise. There are different views about this and they point to different qualities. Psychologists have for some time studied the cognitive bases of expertise and many of these bases have been applied in crucial ways by researchers in artificial intelligence. Computational expert systems seek largely to model human problem-solving abilities. What is important is the overwhelmingly instrumental or procedural nature of expertise that emerges: "Experts solve complex problems considerably faster and more accurately than novices do" (Larkin et al. 1980: 1335).

Similarly, several common features characterize the progression to expertise:

- Learn and apply basic rules.
- Generalize the rules.
- Develop concepts and additional rules.
- Evaluate and assimilate many situations and cases.
- Apply experience and synthesize. (Hankins 1987: 303)[8]

Thus the novice who would be expert learns the procedural *skills* that have already been mastered by experts. This emphasis on procedure does not overlook content; it just gives it a smaller role.

Sociologists shift the focus from a person's skill to his or her standing in a scientific community. This standing or reputation is the result of a vast, multi-articulated system of publications, citations in the literature, awards, appointments and so forth (Garfield 1979; cf. Chubin 1976).

Eugene Garfield cites several studies that purport to demonstrate the expert status of Nobel Prize winners by virtue of the fact that they were more frequently cited in their respective literatures than non-prize winners. The affirmation of expertise as such is only tacit in the citation approach, but the implication is clear: Solid work by good or expert scientists is recognized. In any event, Garfield is aware of potential shortcomings of the approach and says of citation counts that "They very definitely are an interpretive tool that calls for thoughtful and subtle judgments on the part of those who employ them" (p. 249).

Of course, this has the effect of starting us off on a circle as vast as the citation network itself – for who picks the Nobel Prize winners if not scientists who we hoped were affirmed *independently* as experts? Garfield mentions one study that assessed "the accuracy of citation counts as a measure of quality in the field of psychology by asking a panel of experts to list the people who they felt had made the most significant contribution to their specialties" (p. 64). Of course, the "experts" confirmed that the most-often cited work was of the highest quality. The appeal to the panel of experts is as simple and straightforward as it is circular and regressive.

also say something about *clinical experience*, which concept will vex us in subsequent chapters when it is proffered as a foil or kind of counterargument to practice guidelines and the other instantiations of an evidence-based philosophy. Similarly, a definition that is somehow *patient-centered* will help to clarify that the reason to go to all this trouble is not epistemic purity, political correctness or medical fashion; it is because there are good reasons to believe that health care is improved if it is evidence based. Here is what we are getting at, more or less:

Evidence-based medicine . . . is the integration of best research evidence with clinical expertise and patient values.[11] (Sackett et al. 2000: 1).

To be sure, this will require a little unpacking, but it will not go as well as we would like:

By *best research evidence* we mean clinically relevant research, often from the basic sciences of medicine, but especially from patient-centered clinical research into the accuracy and precision of diagnostic tests (including the clinical examination), the power of prognostic markers, and the efficacy and safety of therapeutic, rehabilitative, and preventive regimens. New evidence from clinical research both invalidates previously accepted diagnostic tests and treatments and replaces them with new ones that are more powerful, more accurate, more efficacious, and safer. (Sackett et al. 2000: 1)

This is a good start, but imperfect. We might have "clinically relevant research" but it might be of low quality; this would occasion no disappointment except that we are parsing a definition relying on "best research evidence." Put differently, the concept of "best (research) evidence" should eventually tell us something about what makes it the best. That the research covers a lot of ground does not mean it is any good, let alone the best. The debate over evidence often turns not on how to separate the wheat from the chaff, but how to separate the good wheat from lesser grains. To continue:

By *clinical expertise* we mean the ability to use our clinical skills and past experience to rapidly identify each patient's unique health state and diagnosis, their individual risks and benefits of potential interventions, and their personal values and expectations. (Sackett et al. 2000: 1)

This is the direction we want, but it seems to be conflating "clinical expertise" with "clinical skill." The question of expertise, as we saw in a somewhat different context, does not lend itself to facile appropriation; do not appeal to experts unless you are certain you know what you are getting into. At any rate, surely we do not want to insist of clinicians that they be experts before they can adopt an evidence-based practice. On the contrary, we should want the adoption of an evidence-based practice to be a requirement of all clinicians, and we want this to begin with students. (Of course, it might be that Sackett et al. would reply that by "expertise" they mean "excellence" or "aptitude" or something else that might be demanded of all clinicians and trainees.) Moving on:

> By *patient values* we mean the unique preferences, concerns and expectations each patient brings to a clinical encounter and which must be integrated into clinical decisions if they are to serve the patient. (Sackett et al. 2000: 1)

This sets the bar very high, especially if the failure to integrate all these unique preferences, concerns, etc., would entail the failure of evidence-based practice. The advantage of setting the bar high, though, is that the players' failure becomes attributable in larger part to the players themselves and not to the designers of the game. As above, though, a key motivation for making evidence-based medicine patient centered is that it underscores those for whose sake we are toiling so hard.

This definition has a number of virtues, not least of which is that it strives to be comprehensive (although in so doing it encounters a number of difficulties, as pointed out). It is noteworthy that, perhaps because of this comprehensiveness, it is the definition cited in a key US Institute of Medicine report on quality improvement (Committee on Quality of Health Care in America, Institute of Medicine 2001). Like other IOM reports, this one includes a number of recommendations to government authorities. One such, to the US cabinet secretary for Health and Human Services, reads like the voice of Archie Cochrane from beyond the grave. Listen:

> The Secretary of the Department of Health and Human Services should be given the responsibility and necessary resources to establish and maintain a comprehensive program aimed at making scientific evidence more useful and accessible to clinicians and patients. In developing this program, the Secretary should work with federal agencies and in collaboration with professional and health care associations, the academic and research communities, and the National Quality Forum and other organizations involved in quality measurement and accountability. (Sackett et al. 2000: 1)

Actually, Dr. Cochrane would likely have put it somewhat differently, but the point is clear. From progress to communication to evidence to expertise to the recommendation that government itself take responsibility for improving health care, the idea that clinicians might not have available the conceptual tools of the trade becomes a source of moral offense: Ignorance is blameworthy.

Error and evidence

We are, of course, talking about "individual ignorance" of the sort Cochrane was tacitly bemoaning, and which we were discussing earlier. A person has "individual ignorance," recall, when she or he does not know of, or is unaware of, evidence that others *do* know about or are aware of. The distinction between individual and collective ignorance – a simple affair – is mainly that if no-one has evidence to support a particular belief, then it is not blameworthy if you are among them. But if most people have evidence for a belief, and you are not among them, then you are, or should be, in trouble. Failing to stay abreast of progress in one's field becomes a moral failing. Indeed, as we earlier noticed, the duty to stay up to date was identified in antiquity.

The reason for insisting on everything from adequate training to continuing education to government policies on the accessibility of evidence is that we have varying degrees of warrant to believe that without them, people will be hurt, or, rather, will be hurt more frequently than with them.[12] This is especially true of training; it would be absurd if otherwise. It is almost always bad news when people with no training attempt to practice medicine or nursing. Continuing education is also essential for clinical practice. The clinician who allows educational or pedagogic time to stand still as of the moment of completion of a residency program, say, has arranged things so that after a few years his patients are no longer seeing a physician, but visiting a museum. In both these cases – training and continuing education – the reason we insist on obedience, compliance, and fealty is that people are injured, harmed, or suffer other untoward and generally undesirable outcomes. Ignorance leads to error. Error can lead to medical harm. Preventable harms can be morally blameworthy.

But where does evidence-based medicine fit on this continuum? What about the evidence- and outcomes-based practice guidelines? Do we know that use of, or adherence to, guidelines reduces particular errors – or is that we have reason to believe it will improve outcomes, a general measure? This distinction, between error reduction and outcome optimization, captures one of the great tensions in the debate over evidence-based practice. It is, in many respects, a debate as old as any of the health professions, as old as Hippocrates, Paracelsus, or Florence Nightingale; it is a debate that shapes the relationship between epidemiology and public health on the one hand and Mr. Jones's appointment on Tuesday at 2; it is a debate between individual and group, patient and community, specific rights and collective duties. The debate over evidence-based practice is a reprise of one of the oldest conflicts in the history of civilization and rational inquiry: between individual persons on one hand and groups of them on the other. In philosophical ethics, a parallel debate sets a duty-and-rights-based morality against a utilitarianism that defines good itself as good-for-the-community.

The Institute of Medicine report on quality improvement was actually the second on aspects of quality. The first, *To Err is Human: Building a Safer Health System,* addressed aspects of patient safety (Kohn, Corrigan, and Donaldson 2000). The report suggested that adverse events occur in 2.9%–3.7% of US hospitalizations, with 44000–98000 preventable deaths annually, findings that have been contested and disputed (Brennan 2000, Sox and Woloshin 2000). What is striking about the first report is that it says almost nothing about the role of evidence-based practice, about outcomes, about guidelines.

A comprehensive research program that looked at the effect of evidence-based practice on error reduction would be a worthy and interesting project – if we didn't have our hands full already. Having identified the vast amounts of research and the intractable number of publications as overwhelming the poor twenty-first century clinician, we need to set our sights on the various attempts to make good on Archie Cochrane's dictum. This leads to many and interesting attempts to reduce clinicians' empirical fallibility with more and better research. Aimed at rescuing clinicians from messes of information, we have produced a new kind of evidence, and it has the effect of increasing the cognitive and intellectual demands on professionals who take care of sick people. It is by no means clear yet that in the process it has reduced their fallibility.

NOTES

1 This heading appropriates and alters the title of an important early criticism of outcomes research, "What physicians know" (Tanenbaum 1993).
2 Beddoes hired the chemist Humphrey Davy to conduct some of this research. Sir

Humphrey and some friends, including the poet Samuel Taylor Coleridge, acquired the taste for self-experimentation using nitrous oxide. (Coleridge was of course later to come to depend on opium.) The investigations inspired the conservative Edmund Burke to accuse Beddoes' laboratory of encouraging atheism and sympathy for the French Revolution (Tuttle 1995). It required another half-century before nitrous oxide would be used for anesthesia in dentistry (Abbot 1983, cited by Diemente and Campbell 1983).

3 Louis' evidence was, alas, this: He did not compare patients who were bled against those who were not; rather, he compared those who came to the hospital early in the course of their malady, and were therefore bled early, to those who came late and were bled late. "More of the patients who were bled early died. This comparison between two noncomparable prognostic groups would be completely unacceptable today. Also, the tables in the original text contain some disturbing arithmetic mistakes" (Vandenbroucke 1998: 2001).

4 Note though the suggestion that the reason the British Medical Research Council randomized pulmonary tuberculosis patients in the key 1948 trial was not so much for methodological, empirical, or scientific reasons but to save physicians the difficulty of deciding which patients should receive one of the limited doses of streptomycin (Yoshioka 1998).

5 This article is contained in a delightful collection, *The Origins of Specialization in American Medicine*, edited by the medical historian Charles Rosenberg (1909).

6 Philosophers have sometimes turned to experts as sources of epistemological arbitration (see Putnam 1970).

7 It is even possible to consider that expert opinion itself could be counted as data for evidence-based practice (cf. Ross 2000). We will, in Chapter 2, appeal to the work of the philosopher John Hardwig, whose work on epistemic dependence makes appeal to reliance on scientific experts.

8 Hankins' title is "The paradox of expertise," the paradox being borrowed from Johnson (1983) and concerns the mature expert's inability to remember what it was to be a novice. Note that Johnson, too, gives a strongly instrumental definition of "expert": "An expert is a person who, because of training and experience, is able to do things the rest of us cannot . . ." (p. 78).

9 Moral expertise presents, for some thinkers, a distinct class of issues. This is sometimes related to claims about the (non)existence of moral truths. At any rate, the same confusions we are concerned with here seem to apply in the moral realm (see Burch 1974; Tiles 1984; Baylis 1989; Caplan 1989).

10 Discovering statistical flaws and other failures of peer review has become a growth industry (cf. McGuigan 1995; Welch and Gabbe 1996; Porter 1999).

11 Cf. "Evidence-based clinical practice is an approach to decision making in which the clinician uses the best evidence available, in consultation with the patient, to decide upon the option which suits that patient best" (Muir Gray 1997: 9). This of course

invites rejoinder from critics of, say, culturally sensitive practice in which folk health beliefs must be incorporated into clinical practice. It might be that a patient has false beliefs such that one cannot always give the beliefs serious scientific consideration and hope simultaneously to "suit that patient best." I am thinking, of course, of cases in which the patient is dead as a result of acting (or not acting) on his or her false belief.

12 Virginia Sharpe and Alan Faden consider the relation between error and evidence in a discussion about "the concept of appropriateness in patient care" (Sharpe and Faden 1998).

2

The research synthesis revolution

When this common sense of interest is mutually express'd, and is known to both, it produces a suitable resolution and behaviour. And this may properly enough be call'd a convention or agreement betwixt us, tho' without the interposition of a promise; since the actions of each of us have a reference to those of the other, and are perform'd upon the supposition, that something is to be perform'd on the other part. Two men, who pull the oars of a boat, do it by an agreement or convention, tho' they have never given promises to each other.

David Hume (1739: 541–2)

A special challenge for evidence-based medicine is what to do with all the evidence – all the often confusing, sometimes contradictory, generally hard-to-understand evidence. As science grows, so grows the need to collate, synthesize, and otherwise make sense of a burgeoning corpus. Our task in this chapter is to continue the discussion begun in Chapter 1 and look at a quarter-century of effort to bring together disparate kinds of empirical data and render them useful in practical decision making. It will include a discussion of the conceptual problems that arise when we gather information about the world and use this information to increase understanding and guide decision making. Indeed, the very idea of evidence in medicine is sometimes taken to be a simple matter of linking up facts for the sake of problem solving. But in identifying reasons for our beliefs we also want to know how strong a warrant they provide: how good are the reasons and how good must they be to compel us to revise our beliefs?

Scientific publishing

Suppose a sociopathic hermit who happens to be a brilliant immunology investigator discovers a cure for AIDS. Such a discovery should be cause for much celebration. Our investigator, however, is a hermit because of his preference for solitude and his disdain for human company and convention; he lives in the woods. Moreover, recall, he is a sociopath, which means he actually is malignly disposed to the society from which he has absented himself.

Because he cannot directly harm the society he reviles, yonder, his only hope for gratification of this awful desire is to effect harm indirectly. He can do this quite easily by withholding his great discovery, by keeping it a secret. He harms by willful inaction.

Nowadays, of course, many scholars withhold their results from a larger audience, at least for a while (Chalmers 1990, Blumenthal et al. 1997), but they are motivated not by a desire to harm but by somewhat less perverse motives, usually greed or the desire for fame or recognition. Indeed, these motives are much more familiar and common in the sciences, and we would never attribute them to sociopathy, even as the effect of withholding information for these less malign motives might be identical to that of the sociopathic hermit. To be sure, greed is the evil twin of a desire for just deserts, just as lust for fame is the poor relation of the happy hope for some measure of earned recognition. Sorting these out is not our assignment here.

One point raised by the case of the sociopathic hermit is that his motivations and actions are obviously daft, wrongheaded, and perverse. It just does not make any sense that someone would discover a cure for AIDS and keep it secret for any reason (excepting sociopathy or at least preliminary consultations with a patent lawyer). We can identify three reasons why one would normally make public such a discovery:
(1) Moral. The discovery will reduce contagion, suffering, and correlate ills, and humans have affirmative duties to reduce such evils.[1]
(2) Social. The discoverer of a cure for AIDS will win the admiration of:
    (a) other scientists, who are curious to see how it came about, and
    (b) ordinary folk, who will hail the discoverer for making a contribution to the public good.
(3) Financial. There is reason to suppose that the discoverer(s) of a cure for AIDS will enjoy some prosperity; surely many of those who have so far developed and sold existing treatments have made good business of it, even in cases in which the treatments did not work.

The making-public of a scientific discovery, or even of findings or allegations less noteworthy, has come only comparatively recently to be part of a vast and complex network. What we know of as peer review did not evolve until the twentieth century; what we think of as a scientific journal is a creature younger than the oldest human (c. 2002); what we associate with the availability of resources on the World Wide Web is a phenomenon occupying only the most recent moment in the history of science. One wonders how scientists in pre-journal days achieved any emotional traction in disputes over the priority of discovery. Indeed, one might be inclined to attribute to the slowness of communication itself some part of some disputes over priority, except that this does not account for the fertility of debates that continue over rather old issues: Newton, Leibniz and the calculus; Wallace, Darwin and natural selection; Priestley, Lavoisier and oxygen; or even England and France, which fought more heatedly than Adams and Le Verrier over who discovered the planet Neptune. (For discussions of some of these issues, see Engelhardt and Caplan 1987; Bynum, Lock, and Porter 1992; and Martin and Richards 1995.)

Of course, to publish (Lat. *pūblicāre*) is just to *make public,* and late-twentieth and early twenty-first century scientists are not shy about this exercise. If the sociopathic hermit is at one extreme of a continuum, then surely some contemporary investigators are at the other: publication fetishists whose existence is justified by the appearance of their names on journal articles, including, in some cases, articles with which they have only the slimmest acquaintance.

Many scientific articles appear because their authors are incentivized – better, *induced* – to produce them, where these inducements are somewhat removed from those that would emphasize the growth of knowledge, the sharing of findings with colleagues or, say, reducing human suffering or improving life on Earth. This is just to note that much of the scientific literature – perhaps especially the biomedical literature – is as much about waving arms as it is about communicating results. This is a vulgar glut that pollutes the scientific corpus. It thereby tacitly misinforms other investigators, frustrates students, and in some cases deceives the governments, foundations, and other entities that sponsored the research. It would be an interesting project to study whether, how, and to what extent this over-publication harms the people in whose name the research is being conducted. To the extent that refereed publications drive the engine of evidence-based medicine, then, this is a crisis of the greatest magnitude.

That the biomedical corpus is bloated is little disputed. For years, medical journal editors have tried to cleanse the corpus by reducing redundant and fragmented publication,[2] "courtesy" and other forms of underserved authorship, author–investigator conflicts of interest, and so forth (Huth 1986; Susser and Yankauer 1993; International Committee of Medical Journal Editors 1997; Davidoff et al. 2001). Sometimes they seem to be succeeding, sometimes not. It is not clear how this might be measured, except at the edges. For instance, as a sign of the sociological pressures facing some investigators, it has been shown that men publish more than women – but the work of the women is cited more frequently than that of men (Culotta 1993). One might infer from this that men, perhaps under greater pressure to perform, do so, whereas women devote more attention to quality. There might be other interpretations.

One of the happier denouements of this story of professional venality is that publication, authorship, and the ethical issues raised by affixing one's name to a public document are now a firm part of the curriculum for basic scientists in training; it remains for us to make these issues a part of the training of medical and nursing students and young physicians and nurses. Throughout, the message that perhaps should be in the boldest face is that publishing an article involves responsibility and accountability – as well as grants, promotions, and the respect of one's colleagues. Some temptations are, alas, easier than others to resist.

Here, having failed to resist them so far in biomedical research, is what it has come to: some 23 000 biomedical journals . . . more than two million articles published annually . . . 8000 new clinical trials a year . . . 4400 pages or about 1100 articles in the *British Medical Journal* and the *New England Journal of Medicine* annually (Ad Hoc Working Group for Critical Appraisal of the Medical Literature 1987; Olkin 1995).[3] Fortunately, much of this output (funny how we call it "literature"[4]) is not worth the trouble; as well, fortunately, some of it is. Alas, *un*fortunately, it is not a straightforward matter to tell the difference between the two, at least in advance of reading all of it, not that anyone would or could – or that if one could read all of it, could it also be evaluated in a practically useful way? Moreover, our scientific journals themselves are neither impassive nor impartial; political, social, economic, and other distractions shape and color their reports and so, we infer, the inferences drawn from them (Vandenbroucke 1998).

What this suggests is that we are caught in something of an epistemic or communicative pickle. Either:
(1) there is simply too much useful information to process successfully, or
(2) there is not too much information, but it is too difficult to find or separate from that which is not useful, or
(3) purported sources of reliable clinical information are in some way flawed or corrupt, or,
(4) the amount of useful clinical information is tractable and reliable, and there are means for identifying it in the midst of non-useful information.

Point (1) represents a form of skepticism not worth spending much time on here; (2) attempts to label a type of skepticism that might result from the failure of evidence-based medicine to achieve its goals (perversely, a kind of evidence-based skepticism); (3) represents the sort of stance taken by clinicians who dislike the taste of practice guidelines, outcomes measurements, and the other fruits of evidence-based medicine; and (4) is the conceptual foundation of rational practice and policy, the means to vanquish skepticism, the answer without which continuing progress in the health professions is imperiled. That's the one we want.

The skepticism of clinicians is addressed in Chapter 5. Here we should spend some time looking at the tools available to the evidence-based framer and shaper, the means of surveying the vast landscape of biomedical claims and posits and sorting them out properly.

Scientific synthesis and review

Listen to this, from a valuable early contribution to our understanding of research synthesis:

Why do scientists think that new research is better, or more insightful, or more powerful? The underlying assumption must be that new studies will incorporate and improve upon lessons learned from earlier work. Novelty in and of itself is shallow without links to the past. It is possible to evaluate an innovation only by comparisons with its predecessors . . . For science to be cumulative, an intermediate step between past and future research is necessary: synthesis of existing evidence.[5] (Light and Pillemer 1984: 2–3)

We need, in other words, a consistently reliable way to combine or amalgamate the disparate elements in a large corpus. We need a way to pull it all together. This is not news. Such a synthesis is in fact the goal of the traditional review article, customarily by an expert, or at least an authority, in the field. Are the latest studies progressive or not? Do they add to collective knowledge – or bloat the corpus for political, professional, or economic reasons? What does it all mean to someone who has neither the time nor the inclination (and perhaps not the ability) to make sense of scientific change? Well, review articles for a while produced at least the illusion of providing such a service. A good review article gives some history, some news, some commentary, and some "take-home points."[6] Once one is educated in a field, one might, at least in principle, stay up to date by reading nothing more than review articles.

From narrative review to systematic analysis

But there are a number of problems here, and aspects of them were noted in the 1970s by Cochrane in the United Kingdom and Glass in the United States. Most generally, traditional, narrative review articles are often just not very good. They fail in several ways to do what we want:

(1) Reviews are subjective. There are no rules to guide reviewers about measuring or evaluating the quality of the reports they are reviewing. This means that different reviewers might arrive at different conclusions, engendering, instead of resolving, scientific conflict (Light and Pillemer 1984; cf. Oxman and Guyatt 1988).

(2) Reviews are unscientific. Traditional reviewers often sorted through disparate studies and counted the number of studies supporting each side of a contentious issue. Such a strategy has long been known to overlook study design and quality, sample size and effect size (Hedges and Olkin 1980; Mulrow 1987).

(3) Reviews are unsystematic. The point of a narrative review, recall, was to help find what is useful in the midst of lots that is not useful. "A reviewer unarmed with formal tools to extract and summarize findings must rely on an extraordinary ability to mentally juggle relationships among many variables" (Light and Pillemer 1984: 4; cf. Cook et al. 1992). Most reviewers failed, and in any case there was no easy way to distinguish between those who failed and those who succeeded, at least in time to do any good – perhaps before the appearance of the next review on the topic. (Recall that Beddoes and Cochrane wanted their information updated periodically, if not continuously.)

These insights may plausibly be taken to constitute the origin of the research synthesis revolution (cf. Glass and Kliegl 1983). Science needed better ways of keeping its corpus in order and making it easier or more straightforward for users – scientists, students and, as it became increasingly and urgently clear, clinicians and policy makers – to query the corpus and come away with a good sense of what it all meant. Another way to think about this is to underscore that the modern record of scientific change is not merely about arm-waving boffins admiring the heft of each other's CVs. It is about a duty, sometimes individual and sometimes collective, to make meaningful contributions to the scientific corpus and to be ever-mindful that such contributions have consequences; when we do our worst, colleagues' time can be wasted, institutional resources can be squandered, policy can be led astray and people can be hurt.

Systematic reviews

On one account, "Systematic reviews are concise summaries of the best available evidence that address sharply defined clinical questions" (Mulrow, Cook, and Davidoff 1998: 1). They are "scientific investigations in themselves, with pre-planned methods and an assembly of original studies as their 'subjects'" (Cook, Mulrow, and Haynes 1998: 6–7). At ground, the move to synthesis and systematization comes from the stark and simple realization that if we are prepared to insist that scientific rigor must govern the collection of data, then it makes no sense to stop there. Scientific rigor produces good, reliable results because the world is tractable and effable. It is consistent and governed by discoverable rules (or laws), and as we learn how it works we are able to make increasingly accurate predictions (or prognoses).[7] If all this is the case, then it is perverse not to insist that similar rigor be deployed in analyzing and summarizing the data generated by clinical, observational, and other investigations. The inadequacies of narrative reviews left us no choice but to attempt to develop these epistemic engines.

What makes a review systematic is, well, a system for eliminating or reducing bias and subjectivity and for separating what is of little value from that which is of great(er) value. A systematic review, including meta-analyses, has its work cut out for it. Cynthia Mulrow (1995) identifies nine functions and traits. A systematic review should:

(1) Reduce large amounts of information to "palatable pieces for digestion." This calls for a means of data culling without loss of information and, apparently, without cognitive dyspepsia.

(2) Integrate "critical pieces" of information to make them salient to a broad range of investigators, analysts, and users.

(3) Be efficient. Continuous updating of reviews "can shorten the time between medical research discoveries and clinical implementation of effective diagnostic or treatment strategies."[8]

(4) Demonstrate or establish the generalizability of the studies being synthesized. Different study designs, inclusion criteria, etc., create diversity when what is wanted is some measure of homogeneity.

(5) Assess consistency of relationships. If there is a consistent or regular correlation between treatment and effect, a good systematic review should find it.

(6) Explain inconsistencies and conflicts among data. The converse of (5), this function holds systematic reviews responsible for making sense of inconsistencies in the data.

(7) Increase the power of the analysis by increasing the sample size.
(8) Estimate effect with increased precision. In the streptokinase study cited in note 8, two of the largest trials conformed to already established efficacy evidence, but they "increased precision by narrowing the confidence intervals slightly" (Mulrow 1995).
(9) Improve accuracy, at least in principle.

This is clearly asking a great deal. It requires that the systemizer take large amounts of disparate and sometimes low-quality information, analyze or otherwise process it, and produce conclusions that give us warrant to say we know more than we used to. If all goes well, human suffering is reduced, mortality is delayed, and life is improved.

Meta-analysis

While all meta-analyses are (more or less) systematic, not all systematic reviews are meta-analyses (Chalmers and Altman 1995). In the mid-1970s, Gene Glass, an educational researcher, published a brief paper which, along with Cochrane's *Effectiveness and Efficiency: Random Reflections on Health Services* a few years earlier, signaled the beginning of a new way of thinking about information in the sciences. Indeed, "Primary, secondary, and meta-analysis of research" (Glass 1976) is arguably one of the most influential papers in the history of science.[9] In a splendid account of the American Educational Research Association lecture in San Francisco in April 1976 that led to the paper, Morton Hunt, who interviewed Glass for his book, writes,

> Glass, then in his mid-thirties and fully aware of the topic's potential importance, had labored and agonized over the paper for two years, during which, he recently said, "I was a basket case." But Glass, who describes himself as a highly competitive person, stepped cockily to the podium and with seeming self-assurance gave a lucid, witty, and persuasive talk. The audience [according to one observer] was "blown away by it. There was tremendous excitement about it; people were awestruck." (Hunt 1997: 12)

To observe that the talk and paper have been influential is not to say that they and their progeny have been met with universal praise. (One might be blown away, excited and awestruck, but negatively so.)

In the intervening quarter-century, meta-analysis has become a staple of medical research, as well as those sciences which first embraced it: social science and psychology, management and marketing, education, and epidemiology. Indeed, if the first hearts, if not the first minds, were captured in psychology, educational research, and other social sciences, biomedical scientists eventually outstripped their colleagues and at one point in the 1990s were publishing about twice the number of meta-analyses as social scientists (Bausell et al. 1995). But the embrace, or at least acceptance, of meta-analysis has not been universal. Indeed, it has been reviled, sometimes vehemently. As methodological disputes go, it is a lovely little war, and it puts clinicians in a tight spot: If a method is methodologically controversial, then on what grounds should it be adopted or disdained?

Meta-analysis combines data across sources, which can be clinical trials, observational studies, or even individual patient records. In trying to bypass the narrative review, meta-analysts encountered a number of problems of their own, and these problems, instead of reducing scientific uncertainty about the efficacy of particular treatments and interventions, shifted that uncertainty to the research method itself. If a clinician could be honestly confused about what to make of apparently contradictory studies, meta-analysis sometimes (perhaps often) left them confused about a different set of claims and analyses in the biomedical literature.

We will return to and highlight these questions in Chapter 3. For now, we need only observe that meta-analysis is a tool for attempting to make sense of disparate data; it was and is a vital foot soldier in the research synthesis revolution.

"Levels of evidence"

Here is where we stand. Our attempts, since antiquity, to increase medical knowledge, have succeeded dramatically. We have lots of knowledge. In fact, we have more than we know what to do with. We even have some beliefs that we reckon falsely constitute knowledge, and which must eventually be discarded. This means we should develop some strategy for sifting, organizing, collating, and arranging all this knowledge (which, by the way, no single human can do in his or her head). Moreover, the vague phrase "lots of knowledge" masks the fact that much of what we know is probabilistic, that is, is more-or-less likely to be true, or true given certain circumstances, or true only if we assume that certain conditions are met, or *generally* true. Further, we seek medical knowledge in part – perhaps in large part – to change the world. This requires that we have some adequate mechanism for communicating or disseminating what we know, else clinicians would not know what to do.

From research and observation to collection and storage to analysis and synthesis to dissemination and communication to application and practice (which provide data for more research . . .), this is the great chain of clinical practice – the circle of clinical life. At its conceptual center is evidence or, perhaps too often, statements, posits, and reckonings which are mistaken for evidence but which are either false, misguided, or proffered too quickly or too early. If evidence-based care is the grail of contemporary health practice, then "evidence lite" is surely its bane. So, the research synthesis revolution we are considering would not make any sense if it did not attempt to help us sort out the nine putative functions and traits of a systematic review, given variations in the reliability and quality of the material being reviewed systematically. How, in other words, ought we assign value to the different kinds or levels of evidence? To rephrase as a question the challenge presented in Chapter 1, and which lies at the center of our inquiry: *How should we make decisions in the face of scientific uncertainty?* Further: Under what circumstances, if any, is error morally blameworthy? How does the fallibility of our science affect judgments of blameworthiness?

One effort to address the problem of the variable quality or reliability of evidence attempts to rank "levels of evidence" according to different aspects of clinical practice, including therapy, prognosis, diagnosis and economic and decision analysis.

What are we to do when the irresistible force of the need to offer clinical advice meets with the immovable object of flawed evidence? All we can do is our best: give the advice, but alert the advisees to the flaws in the evidence on which it is based. (Phillips et al. 2001)

The Oxford Centre for Evidence-based Medicine does this by stratifying levels of evidence based on degrees of methodological power and leverage.[10] So the lowest level of evidence is "expert opinion without critical appraisal . . ." and the highest level is shared by systematic reviews of randomized controlled trials, individual randomized controlled trials (with narrow confidence intervals), or "all-or-none" observational data in which either all patients die before a treatment is available but, later, some survive when the treatment becomes available, or some died before the treatment's availability but none die on the treatment. This has intuitive heft, makes perfect sense, and, indeed, seems to (be trying to) meet a vital need. So what's wrong, or missing?

The movement for evidence-based practice is in some respects a victim of its own success. The demands of evidence-based medicine are so straightforward and so reasonable that we have come to think that meeting them will be a straightforward matter as well. There are several things wrong with this view (each to be elaborated somewhat more in Chapters 3 and 5). First, look again at the topmost level of the scale (systematic reviews, trials with narrow confidence intervals, and all-or-none data). Grouping evidence thus has the effect of broadening the "gold standard" for biomedical evidence, displacing the randomized control trial as alone in its excellence. Indeed, this strategy swallows trials whole, but it leaves unresolved the important debate over the relation between trials and systematic reviews in the first place: Does one acquire tidier, better, or more evidence by systematically reviewing a cluster of trials – or by conducting a new, well designed, and very large trial? Second, as perhaps it must, the levels-of-evidence tool is careful not to overpromise.[11] That is, a disclaimer makes it clear that the levels "speak only to the validity of the evidence about prevention, diagnosis, prognosis, therapy, and harm," and that other tools "must be applied to the evidence to generate clinically useful measures of its potential clinical implications and to incorporate vital patient-values into the ultimate decisions." It is, in part, a reminder at the core of the enterprise that no mere algorithm will be completely adequate to the task. The third point is partly terminological and, again, less a comment on this particular tool than on the evidence-based firmament. In the middle of the scale one encounters "outcomes research," which is not defined in the site's glossary, but which we may take to mean those studies, often hospital based, that are based on reviews of patient charts and which are often used to assess quality of care and to try to achieve error reduction. There is no clear theoretical underpinning for these chart reviews, even as they are assigned ever greater roles in matters ranging from infection control to evaluation and approval by accrediting bodies. The point for our purposes now is that to allow one's practice to be shaped by "outcomes research" is apparently thought by many (at least in North America) to be or to *constitute* evidence-based practice. While there is no doubt that chart reviews and outcomes research produce evidence, they are on no account necessary or sufficient to support claims of evidence-based practice. (See Muir Gray (1997) and Sharpe and Faden (1998) for discussions of some of these issues.)

All this is, in some respect, to bear witness to the early stages of a transformation in clinical practice in which we try to match the realization of the inadequacy of our evidentiary warrants to new tools for improving or increasing those warrants. As we will see in greater detail in Chapter 3, one of the greatest and most interesting challenges is to accomplish this without falling into a regress such that every attempt to improve evidence is itself subject to dispute about its evidentiary support.

Toward systematic research synthesis

We began this chapter with a thought experiment about a sociopathic hermit who discovered a cure for AIDS but kept it under wraps. We have moved from there to the duty to publish to the duty to be aware of what is published to the duty to incorporate those facts, that evidence, into one's practice. Moreover, these duties – and there are a great deal of them, aren't there? – are not likely to be met by delegation or assignment. The clinician cannot say to an assistant, "Please evaluate those materials, yonder, and, as appropriate, learn about them for me. Then ensure that I act in accordance with them. Thanks . . ." To the extent that hewing to a scientific standard of care is a moral obligation, this is just another way of making the point trumpeted in all introductions to ethics for new medical and nursing students: *All clinical decisions have ethical components.* It might be that they are obvious or trivial or not worth belaboring, but they are there nonetheless. It follows that attending to quality, error avoidance, and the like are also moral imperatives.

Now, the busy clinician has a number of responses, not all of them snide or angry. First, he or she might demand (as if an interrogatory statement carried its own answer, especially the one favored by the interrogator), "Am I a physician or a librarian? I have neither the time nor the inclination nor the skill to monitor and evaluate all you say I must in order to meet my many obligations." Or words to that effect. Another protest might be on methodological grounds and might make the case that *no-one* is able to do all that is required, that is, it is not a question of time, inclination, or skill but, rather, that the task required cannot be obligatory because it is impossible for any individual to complete it. If no-one can do the duty, then it violates the 1600-year-old principle in moral philosophy that "ought implies can."[12] The proponents of evidence-based practice say that it is precisely the many demands on the contemporary clinician that make the evidence-based stance so useful, if not necessary.

Something broader is needed. It will not do to respond to those who are agnostic or skeptical about evidence that the evidence-based movement is the solution to their problems because it does all the hard work, the heavy lifting. What is wanted is a systemic justification for the system – a theoretical foundation to justify acting on beliefs for which we have second- and third-hand warrant but no direct reason. Put another way, the busy clinician needs not only research synthesis but a good reason to suppose that the results of complex (and perhaps inscrutable) statistical analysis should be incorporated in the clinic, that the latest systematic review will improve care of today's patients, that disparate data can inform health policy when the stakes are high. We want it to be rational to question or challenge authority but irrational to discard collective wisdom.

Communities of inquirers and epistemic interdependence

The American philosopher Charles Sanders Peirce (1839–1914) contended that it is not individual scientists who know, but instead a *community of inquirers*. Indeed, science depends on communities, on *cooperation by members* of communities:

Science is to mean for us a mode of life whose single animating purpose is to find out the real truth, which pursues this purpose by a well-considered method, founded on thorough acquaintance with such scientific results already ascertained by others as may be available, and which seeks cooperation in the hope that the truth may be found, if not by any of the actual inquirers, yet ultimately by those who come after them and who shall make use of their results . . . Science being essentially a mode of life that seeks cooperation, the unit science must, apparently, be fit to be pursued by a number of inquirers. (Peirce 1958: 7.54–7.55; cf. 5.311, 5.316)

This requires that members of the community care about what is known – one cannot absent oneself from the hunt in hopes that the absence will not be missed later, when the bird is cooked and the wine is being poured. This does not mean that physicians all need to become scientists, investigators, trialists, researchers . . . only that they follow the debates, attend to and care about the results, and *think* about what is best for patient care. With such an approach they will be better able and better prepared to trust those colleagues who are doing the number crunching. It turns out that this trust is necessary if clinical science is to progress.

The contemporary philosopher John Hardwig has done an outstanding job in making sense of the "fact that I believe more than I can become fully informed about" (Hardwig 1985: 340). From physics to biology to mathematics we are not able to do all the experiments that inform our beliefs, not able to understand all the concepts involved, unable even to communicate the news of scientific change such that a colleague would be irrational to doubt it. Hardwig is ultimately appealing to reliance on experts so that we might be able to know "vicariously" through them; it is a strategy that goes against the grain of what he calls "epistemological individualism" (ibid: 339).[13] Further, Hardwig develops the links between research integrity and knowledge by exploring the grounds a nonexpert has for believing an expert:

> Modern knowers cannot be independent and self-reliant, not even in their own fields of specialization. In most disciplines, those who do not trust cannot know; those who do not trust cannot have the best evidence for their beliefs. In an important sense, then, trust is often epistemologically even more basic than empirical data or logical arguments: the data and the argument are available only through trust. (Hardwig 1991: 693–4)

This intellectual division of labor has a number of virtues. It is fallible; given the probabilistic nature of the evidence in evidence-based medicine, anything less than a robust fallibility will leave us in the lurch. It is comprehensive; we need to justify clinicians' beliefs across a broad domain. And it is intuitively powerful; does one really need to be a molecular biologist to understand that tamoxifen is more successful in treating breast cancer in some genetic subgroups than others? (King et al. 2001). Indeed, the idea of an epistemic division of labor seems precisely what is needed to help make evidence simultaneously accessible to ordinary clinicians and to prevent it from being parodied as providing (mere) cookbooks or algorithms. We will need to return to these themes throughout this book, and they will serve us well in conclusion in Chapter 7.

There is also an unavoidable, but fortunately delicious, sense here in which the World Wide Web becomes necessary as a medium for supporting this epistemic dependence and division of labor. A clinician at a computer (in principle) anywhere can (in principle) search and sort and digest (in principle) a vast amount of information. By these means, clinicians take responsibility for their own information needs and even raise questions about the need for medical publishing as we know it (LaPorte et al. 1995). Well, we do not need to expect or hope for the demise of the medical journal, although if we have learned anything so far it is that scientific communication and the tools for gathering data to help revisit and revise beliefs are themselves subject to evolution and change. The medical student or scholar is as likely to be looking at a journal at home on a computer screen as at the library in a carrel stacked with journals. Surely nothing aside from truth, quality, and tradition . . . and perhaps esthetics . . . constitutes adequate reasons to prefer the one over the other.

We began this chapter with a motto – a quotation from David Hume – who, in making a point about morality, regarding "agreement or convention," should equally be seen to be urging us to reflect on customs of sharing. The rowers must presume each other's good will, common purpose, and dedication. The strategy will be the same for a lunch at a lakeside or a rescue from a shipwreck. It is when the stakes are highest, of course, that morality places on us the greatest duties.

NOTES

1 On one important account of morality, irrationality itself is defined as desiring evils such as pain or death. Professor Bernard Gert's system of moral rules and ideals (Gert 1998) links rationality, morality, and the consequences of human action in a way that captures nicely the moral intuitions that shape the debates over, among other issues, scientific publication and authorship.

2 This includes the fragmentation of study reports into what has come to be known as the "least publishable unit" (Broad 1981).

3 According to the working group, the two million articles would form a 500-meter stack. We can add to the calculation by noting that if you wanted to keep up with your journals and were to take only 1 day's holiday during the year (Gutenberg's birthday, say) and did nothing – *nothing* – other than read journals, you would have to make your way through 228.93 articles per hour to complete your awful task (cf. Davidoff et al. 1995).

4 Much medical writing is just poor: "If we could get the citation seekers out of our journals and into peer-reviewed electronic databases, we could rid ourselves of their vernacular and start to share our ideas in a clear, honest, and interesting way" (O'Donnell 2000: 491). It would indeed be interesting to study the effects (on quality? cost? outcomes?) of bad writing.

5 Note that the growth of the research synthesis movement in the 1970s and 1980s was driven largely by psychology, education studies, and corrections and somewhat less by biomedical science. (cf. Pillemer and Light (1980), and the early literature on meta-analysis, to be discussed shortly and in Chapter 3).

6 The very idea of a "take-home point" seems to come from medical education and it is used in the following kind of context: a lecture provides background, news and commentary – but what busy clinicians want and need is not the delicious details and

reasons that so excite educators and other intellectuals, but just the distilled bits of news that can be clinically deployed. Compare in this regard the use of "clinical pearls," or tools or practices that seem consistently to work and, in medical publishing, the increasing use of "key point" summaries and abstracts, itemized "what you should know" blurbs and pull-out boxes that are, it is to be hoped, not intended to substitute for reading the full report but which, one fears, are used as substitutes for reading and understanding the full report. In fact, reliance on abstracts and summaries has inspired research into the content of abstracts themselves, with less-than-happy results: Abstracts have been found to be less informative and consistent than needed (Hayward et al. 1993), and – even in the case of reports of practice guidelines – too often do not accurately reflect the research articles they are summarizing (Pitkin, Branagan, and Burmeister 1999).

7 These are among the core beliefs of scientific realists or universalists, who are opposed by scientific anti-realists or relativists. This philosophical debate originates with the Greek Sophist Protagoras who argued (unsuccessfully in Plato's *Protagoras*) that "Man is the measure of all things." That the world is (more or less) knowable, consistent and predictable is little in dispute among physicians. We may hypothesize that even the most committed anti-realists would not prefer someone of like (epistemological) mind to perform neurosurgery, treat advanced heart disease, or manage their child's cancer.

8 Mulrow here cites Lau et al. (1992), a review of 33 trials which showed that intravenous streptokinase for myocardial infarction could have been shown to be life saving years before the treatment was submitted to, and approved by, the United States' Food and Drug Administration.

9 Glass here coined the term "meta-analysis" and used the term "effect size" to signify a standardized mean difference – so some of the influence is doubtless terminological (see Olkin (1990) for a taut introduction to meta-analytic history).

10 The origin of the effort was a quarter-century ago with the Canadian Task Force on the Periodic Health Examination (1979). The Web-based levels-of-evidence project began in 1998 and is updated periodically. It is part of "The EBM Toolbox," an outstanding resource that provides "an assortment of materials which are very useful for practitioners of EBM." The site is available at http://cebm.jr2.ox.ac.uk/docs/toolbox.html.

11 This second point is not so much a comment on the Oxford Centre as such (neither is it a criticism) as an observation about its need to hedge its bets. It is a wise and forthright disclaimer, and all evidence-based efforts need to evaluate this approach. Indeed, many do.

12 The idea that it is nonsensical to require people to do things unless they actually are able to do them is attributed to Pelagius, a fifth-century figure famous as much for having antagonized Augustine with his notion as for the notion itself. Augustine reckoned that the concept could not be reconciled with (his view of) original sin.

13 Here is how it works: Suppose *A* is an expert, *B* a layperson and *p* a scientific proposition. *A* believes that *p*. Is that a good reason for *B* to believe that *p*? ". . . I think we
must say that *B*'s belief is rationally justified – even if he does not know or understand
what *A*'s reasons are – if we do not wish to be forced to conclude that a very large percentage of beliefs in any complex culture are simply and unavoidably irrational or
nonrational. For, in such cultures, more is known that is relevant to the truth of one's
beliefs than anyone could know by himself. And surely it would be paradoxical for
epistemologists to maintain that the more that is known in a culture, the less rational the beliefs of individuals in that culture" (Hardwig 1985: 339). Hardwig's view
here (especially at p. 337, note 1) seems to cohere nicely with technical aspects of
Peter Achinstein's important account (Achinstein 1978).

3

Evidence of evidence, and other conceptual challenges

I have little patience with scientists who take a board of wood, look for its thinnest part and drill a great number of holes where drilling is easy.   Albert Einstein[1]

In less than a quarter-century, efforts to combine or amalgamate the results of diverse research projects have become ubiquitous. Meta-analysis, for instance, has found employment in psychology and psychotherapy, social science, education, meteorology, marketing, management and business studies, and, perhaps especially, in medicine and epidemiology, including genetics and all aspects of clinical trials, drug efficacy, disease prevention, investigator education and reporting, public health, health policy, and patient education and behavior. This chapter addresses the notion of "meta-evidence" by looking at its relation to causation and rational clinical belief. Research synthesis and systematic science raise vitally important methodological and conceptual questions and so the chapter will also identify key methodological controversies and criticisms provoked by meta-analysis and other systematic reviews. What kind of scientific evidence is a meta-analysis or a systematic review, and how best should these tools be incorporated in research and clinical practice?

Evidence

Evidence is information that we use in deciding whether to believe a statement or proposition. It bears on the truth of our beliefs. A proposition might very well be true, but if there is no evidence that points in that direction, then there is no reason to believe it to be true. This is partly what is meant by *rationality*, which demands reasons for holding beliefs, and is related to the issue we encountered in Chapter 1 in the discussion about the percentage of medicine that is evidence based: A physician might be right without having adequate reason to think so. When such a physician has a good outcome we should regard this as *therapeutic luck*. There are all kinds of evidence and, indeed, many kinds of information can constitute evidence depending on the proposition whose truth we are after. The histories of science and philosophy are intertwined about the axis of evidence, each using and appealing to the other.

Unfortunately, information does not always bear a direct or simple relation to the truth of propositions. It might be that information supports the truth of more than one proposition (or hypothesis or clinical theory[2]), including diagnoses, prognoses, and treatment plans, and these may be incompatible. The patient who says, "It hurts here, a lot," may be giving information that bears on the truth of a diagnosis of "perforated ulcer," "appendicitis," or "trauma caused by domestic violence." There is just not (yet) enough information to decide which is correct. (In this way, one can have evidence for a false proposition.) Signs, symptoms, and reports of signs and symptoms are eminently local phenomena, but are no less evidence for that. This is why we teach students the importance of physical examination. It is also why we teach the importance of making differential diagnoses: different diagnoses suggest different approaches to, and strategies for, collecting more information, with the hope of turning that information into evidence.[3]

In Chapter 1 it was mentioned that having evidence does nothing to help address the question of quality. One might have limited or poor evidence, or even unlimited poor evidence. On even the most cursory glance through old medical journals and texts, one is struck by how much information was available to support propositions now known to be false. And anyone who has missed a diagnosis knows that awful feeling – that awful epistemological feeling – that comes from having had many reasons to accept as true something later found to be false. Such reasons, and perhaps all of them, are inconclusive, by which is meant that belief in empirical propositions is fallible. There is no solace for the skeptic or relativist here, however – only eventual disappointment for dogmatists.

Observations, tests, and experiments

Clinicians and scientists share a number of duties, even if the clinician does no research and the scientist sees no patients. There is a sense in which every patient is a kind of experiment or, rather, an opportunity to do some applied science. To learn what ails Patient P, one might make a number of *observations*, conduct a number of *tests*, and even perform a number of little *experiments*. (Medical language sometimes renders the undertaking of these experiments as "treating the patient empirically" . . . what this seems to mean is that a patient is provided with a drug or other intervention to see if it works.)

A biomedical scientist also makes observations, which might or might not be of patients themselves, or their cells, tissues, or other parts, using various instruments to aid the sense perceptions; conducts tests, as with stains, reagents, temperature change, and so on; and performs experiments. Now, these experiments can range from extremely small or local studies to enormous, randomized, double-blind, placebo-controlled trials. We sometimes use the term "study" to cover all this information elicitation, whether it be by a laboratory scientist, an epidemiologist, or a clinical trial investigator.

As we move from observation to test to trial, we are seeking to improve the quality (or reduce the error) of each form of information elicitation. While an observation can provide important information, it is also susceptible to numerous perceptual and other errors and biases. If we must acknowledge the fallibility and corrigibility of our observations – and we must – then even a clinician with great powers of observation might, at the end of a long career, be completely mistaken about what he or she has been observing. This is, in part, the impetus for the evolution of clinical trials over the past half-century or so: Systematically organizing observations and systematically challenging living organisms reduces bias and therefore error, and therefore produces more useful information, and therefore more reliable evidence, and therefore greater warrant for our beliefs.[4] This is the essence of rational decision making in biomedical science.

But even our best tools for reducing bias fail to eliminate it; and some of these tools even present new sources of bias. This – coupled with the facts that (1) nature gives up its secrets slowly and not always in a stepwise, orderly fashion, and (2) human variation introduces aspects of great complexity into the business of biomedical discovery – means that even our best evidence will be inconclusive in many cases, and always probabilistic. We sometimes want the world to be simple, and it fails to comply. We apparently want our studies to point in a direct and unambiguous way to a set of beliefs, when the task that is actually before us requires that we use critical judgment to make inferences based on our observations, tests, and experiments. I am reminded of the young investigator whose protocol was being vetted by an institutional review board (or research ethics committee). The protocol design was faulted for not including enough subjects to achieve statistical significance. The young investigator responded, "That's OK – we just want to see if it works before trying it on a lot of people."[5]

Meta-evidence

Observations, tests, and experiments are usually made or performed on physical objects or entities, including people.[6] In the biomedical sciences, investigators carry out a great many such inquiries with the effect, as we saw in Chapter 2, that writers of narrative reviews are generally unable to make reliable sense out of it all, at least for some lines of inquiry. The results of some experiments point in one direction, some in the other, and some nowhere at all. This is a problem if the goal of the inquiry is, say, to learn which of two compounds is more likely to save the lives of heart or cancer or infectious disease patients. At any rate, narrative reviews are judged to be subjective, unscientific, and unsystematic. The narratives are biased, not (necessarily) because of any intellectual shortcoming, scientific confusion, or economic conflict but because the nature of the review itself was such that reviewers could not find an Archimedean or neutral vantage point from which to survey the vast holdings of the house of science.

Among the responses to this unacceptable state of affairs – unacceptable because it constitutes a surrender to the forces of error and skepticism – is the movement to make such reviews themselves scientific. The goal of founding and grounding a logic of the systematic review has, in about a quarter of a century, led to a transformation in our ideas about evidence. Consider briefly that the first (and by some lights the best) form or kind of evidence is that produced by human sensory apparatuses. Our observations, auscultations, olfactions, and so on provide a more or less reliable stream of information about the world. This information might be very simple ("bright," "loud," "salty") or quite complex, depending on the kind of entity or event producing the sense data. Indeed, there is much important philosophical work to be done here, and philosophers have been doing it since Plato. But except for the most fatuous skeptic, relativist, solipsist, or idealist, there are few good reasons to doubt that our sense impressions are in some way caused by the *world*.[7] Our sensations are *about* the world, more or less. So when we allow this sensory information to guide us in deciding whether to believe some statement or other, we are making a judgment about the way the world is; the judgment is based on a causal relationship between the world and the human sensorium.

That causal relationship is a cornerstone of human knowledge. But when we aggregate evidence from several sources (each of which is based on an ensemble of causal relationships), our aggregation or pooling produces information that is no longer directly about the world. It is information about other evidence. It is therefore at least one causal level removed from the phenomena it is purportedly about.

Causation and causal relationships

In a tasty understatement, the philosopher Wesley Salmon (1925–2001) observed that "The attempt to gain scientific understanding of the world is a complicated matter" (Salmon 1998: 78). Setting aside consideration of ways in which we might distinguish between scientific and non-scientific understanding of the world, the point in saluting Prof. Salmon is twofold. First, he has done as much as any other contemporary thinker to make sense of the relationship between causation and explanation, where this relationship can inform our understanding of clinical skills in an environment shaped by uncertainty (cf. Salmon 1984). How, for instance, should we try to explain why an intervention works with some patients and not with others – when they all seem to have the same malady, when the intervention's mechanism of action is thought to be well understood, and when there is antecedent reason to believe that the intervention will, in fact, work for all patients? The best answers to these kinds of questions will include details about causal and explanatory relationships. Second, when Prof. Salmon tells us that scientific understanding is complicated, there is a sense in which he hasn't seen anything yet. For if it is complicated in dealing with shorter or more directly connected causal chains, then our work is truly cut out for us when links take us from natural phenomena to experiments to re-analysis to a completely new level of scientific inference, evidence, and explanation. The causal chains of research synthesis – chains that shape and warrant our biomedical beliefs – are further removed from the world than the observations and trials that once served exclusively as the cornerstones of clinical decision making. This is not to say that they are false or less reliable; it is to say that we need to re-evaluate some conceptual foundations before building too grand an edifice.

We should make this point from a different perspective. Suppose a clinician were to consider recommending that a heart attack patient receive aspirin therapy to reduce mortality and reinfarction. She would then appeal to what is arguably one of the best-known clinical trials in the history of biomedical research – the "ISIS-2 trial" (the second International Study of Infarct Survival, ISIS-2 1988; cf. Peto, Collins, and Gray 1995.). This experiment showed that aspirin therapy caused a dramatic (20%) reduction in vascular death. It is hence uncontroversial to infer that, in about a fifth of acute myocardial infarction (AMI) patients, aspirin will *inhibit* platelet aggregation, which *reduces* vascular events, which *lowers* mortality. The italicized verbs here point to a causal relationship,[8] a sequence of events, linking the ingestion of aspirin with reduced mortality.

The sequence may be complicated; this is why the study of causation and explanation is so difficult, and rewarding. But we nevertheless are prepared to view the causal chain as direct, at least in some cases, as suggested by (1):

1.   Ingest aspirin > inhibit platelet cyclo-oxygenase > prevent thromboxane A_2 formation > . . . > reduce mortality[9]

We should regard this as the beginning of an explanation of the ISIS-2 results. We see a series of links from aspirin to patients to outcome. The ISIS-2 investigators had before them more than 1000 human patients in the aspirin/placebo group. The chain represented by (1) appears to apply to about 20% of them. Our clinician can recommend aspirin therapy, reasonably secure in the causation-informed belief that about one in five of her post-AMI patients will fare better than they would have had she prescribed no post-AMI therapy. If someone were to ask her *why* she recommends such a course, she can appeal to the links noted in (1).

In a systematic review, the results of several trials are aggregated. We no longer necessarily see the details of *aspirin to patient to outcome*, but rather a series of outcomes that have been aggregated and analyzed. Perhaps we can represent this as in (2):

2.   Study outcome 1 + study outcome 2 + study outcome n → reduce mortality

If (2) could, for the sake of discussion, be made to stand for the work of the Antiplatelet Trialists' Collaboration (1994) meta-analysis, then our clinician has fine warrant to recommend post-AMI aspirin therapy (and others as well). The difference between (1) and (2) is that (1) makes explicit a causal chain (an angle bracket '>' is used to show this) whereas (2) makes no causal claim at all but illustrates an inference (a right arrow '→' is used to illustrate this). In (2), the different trials did not cause their successors and, moreover, nothing in (2) will help the clinician *explain* why she thinks post-AMI aspirin therapy will work – at least not in the same way that (1) does; if someone now asks her *why* she recommends aspirin therapy, her answer will rely not on observations or measurements about the world, but on aggregated and concatenated inferences. The first version of this point was made by the philosopher Ed Erwin who, in a discussion of meta-analysis in psychotherapy, argued that the integration of diverse data erodes the credibility of claims for causal connections between psychotherapy and beneficial therapeutic outcomes (Erwin 1984; cf. Goodman 1998b). The question as to whether investigators have identified causal connections is easier asked, more hotly debated, and, often, more difficult to answer in behavioral medicine and epidemiology than in clinical medicine.

Seeing that an event is more or less consistently followed by another event should increase our confidence that some sort of causal relationship is at work (subject of course to many Humean caveats). Seeing others' *reports* of such a relationship should also increase this confidence, but it is at least one level removed from the object in the world we are studying – or treating. Our clinician's confidence might be based on neither the knowledge that aspirin inhibits the action of platelet cyclo-oxygenase nor that ISIS-2 found as a practical matter that it saved the lives, for a while, of 20% of patients receiving it.[10]

Her belief might be shaped by no explanatory story, and it has no explanatory value. She might not even be able to say why she has come to hold it. Strikingly, though, she is correct. Her belief is true. But as we noted a little earlier, it is a belief based on a wholly new kind of evidence.

Meta-analysis and the systematic review

Origins, progress, and challenges

The idea that one might productively combine the results of several studies is generally traced to the British mathematician, statistician, and eugenicist Karl Pearson (1857–1936). Pearson, a protégé of Sir Francis Galton (1822–1911), founded the journals *Biometrika* and *Annals of Eugenics* (now *Annals of Human Genetics*). His book, *National Life From the Standpoint of Science*, aimed in part at saving Britain from those who are "unfit" but reproductively successful: "We have two groups in the community – one parasitic on the other. The latter thinks of tomorrow and is childless, the former takes no thought and multiplies. . . . the parasite will kill its host, and so ends the tale for both alike" (Pearson 1905). Pity. The previous year, Pearson published a paper that is apparently the earliest antecedent of Glass's seminal "Primary, secondary, and meta-analysis of research." Pearson's goal was to sort out evidence for the efficacy of typhoid inoculation, and in "Report on certain enteric fever inoculation statistics" (Pearson 1904), he calculated and averaged the inoculation–mortality correlations reported in five typhoid studies and compared this with effect sizes of inoculations for other diseases.

Nearly a century later, meta-analysis, much refined and enjoying a secondary literature of its own, has been applied to a vast array of human inquiries. These range from agriculture, cosmology, and management to education, genetics, and environmental health. Perhaps its greatest impact has been in psychology, epidemiology, and medicine.[11] In defining his terms, Glass glossed "primary analysis" as "the original analysis of data in a research study. It is what one typically imagines as the application of statistical methods"; "secondary analysis" was given as "the reanalysis of data for the purpose of answering the original research question with better statistical techniques, or answering new questions with old data"; and "meta-analysis" emerged as "nothing more than the attitude of data analysis applied to quantitative summaries of individual experiments" (Glass, McGaw, and Smith 1981: 21).

This is wrong: Meta-analysis is *much* more than "the attitude of data analysis," although its framers should be forgiven the lapse. From the time of the first meta-analysis, every aggregation of studies has served as a kind of unintentional cloaking device to isolate users from the causal chains that informed the "original analysis." As we saw, the reasons meta-analysis evolved – the reasons that science itself demanded the new methods of research synthesis – were that those good-old single studies were either too small, too unclear, too contradictory, and hence too unreliable to be given the last word. Narrative reviews were subjective and conflicted. It might be that individual studies and narrative reviews of them are closer to the ground and therefore more clearly or directly reflect causal processes, but that is in itself inadequate reason to declare victory (or closure) and move on. There is a lot wrong with the gold-standard randomized controlled trial, which we would do well to keep in mind while considering what a complicated matter it is to obtain understanding in the sciences.

Meta-analyses, systematic reviews, pooled analyses, etc.,[12] all consistently raise certain problems and challenges. We need to consider these, for they contribute greatly to the problem we are trying to solve for clinicians, policy makers, and others, namely: *How should one make decisions in the face of scientific uncertainty, especially when human life is on the line?* If evidence-based practice can reduce uncertainty and therefore better inform clinical decisions, then it becomes blameworthy not to bend one's knee at this altar. Anything that impeaches an evidence-based claim, or trivializes the movement, therefore carries a weighty scientific and moral burden. Contrarily, congruently weighty burdens are borne by leaders and soldiers of the evidence-based movement, who, at great scientific and moral peril, might presume closure in complex domains, terminating debate and chilling research in cases where more debate and research are precisely what is wanted.

We need to review several problems with meta-analysis and systematic reviews, some well known and others not. We do this not, like some, in hopes that clinicians will set aside these methods or hold them in low regard but, rather, to clarify the nature of the uncertainty that shapes even the best-informed clinical decision making and so presents clinicians with what may be called their "greatest unacknowledged ethical challenge." We will look at problems related to the data that go into systematic reviews, the explanatory uncertainty and apparent regress that systematic reviews seem to engender, and, last, the practical utility of the reviews (and rely at a number of points on Goodman 1998b).

Problems with biomedical research data and reports

We spent a good deal of time in Chapters 1 and 2 savoring the origins of the evidence-based practice movement and the research synthesis revolution. Along the way we saw that humans are scientifically garrulous – we certainly produce a great many articles and reports – and it is increasingly clear that this corpus, this body of knowledge, this repository we rely on to guide us in countless life-or-death decisions, is actually of inconsistent and sometimes even low quality. So, while biomedical science demands that we use rigorous methods in synthesizing our data, we are sometimes embarrassed by a dirty secret: even with perfect data synthesis and flawless systematic review (whatever these would look like), the stuff being synthesized is sometimes poor, false, misleading, off the mark, or wrong.

This was actually clear well before historical trends "were consolidated and named EBM by a group led by Gordon Guyatt at McMaster University in Canada" (Sackett et al. 2000: 2).[13] It was clear in the work of those who were worried that the process of peer review was faulty, biased, and otherwise flawed . . . It was obvious to those who wanted to make medical care more rational for economic reasons: If a procedure did not work well or often, then why ever should anyone pay for it? . . . And it was clear at the beginning of the quality-in-health-care movement:

> . . . for at least some important practices, the existing evidence is of such poor quality that it is virtually impossible to determine even what effect the practice has on patients, much less whether that effect is preferable to the outcomes that would have occurred with other options. Furthermore, whatever the quality of the existing evidence, our current ability to analyze that information is primitive. As a consequence of these two findings, we simply do not know the appropriate standard of care for some medical practices. (Eddy and Billings 1988: 20; cf. Eddy 1993)

One can systematically review and meta-analyze to one's heart's content, but if (some of) the data being pooled, reviewed, and analyzed are flawed, then it will be quite difficult to say when the research that concerns these activities has been progressive.

There is good news and bad news here, and they are closely intertwined. The bad news is just what we have been debating: Clinical research is (methodologically, statistically, conceptually) flawed and so must be its synthesis, in some degree. But surely the observation that research is flawed, in some degree, should be set against the uncontroversial benefits of biomedical research over the past half-century. Scientific progress can be maddeningly slow and this, like difficult problems in ethics, may gladden the hearts of relativists and skeptics. But the point of Einstein's motto for this chapter is in part that we err badly when we mistake difficulty for intractability or conflate the slowness of an inquiry for the ineffability of the subject of our science.

We sometimes, that is, take too great a delight in the discovery of failure, especially when it blinds us to success. It is said that the only thing worse than finding a worm in an apple is finding half a worm. The good news in such a case is, of course, that not only can we then go about minimizing damage, but we are likely to take greater pains to avoid this unhappy occurrence in the future. The good news represented by the acknowledgment that clinical data and the data from clinical trials are imperfect is that once this shortcoming has been detected, we can set about trying to improve things. This seems to be precisely what has happened. Indeed, meta-analysts have themselves identified errors that perhaps would not have been detected otherwise, or in a timely manner, and "authors of meta-analyses are forever deploring poor quality in studies rather than papering it over with calculations" (Wachter 1988: 1407).

Indeed, the rigor with which controlled trials, for instance, are vetted has itself increased, from a noteworthy early report (Sacks et al. (1987), updated as Sacks et al. (1992), with the authors underscoring the "noticeable improvement" since 1987). We increasingly not only know what to look for, we are better able to know when we have found it, when we have not found it, and the best ways of finding it. It is becoming apparent that systematic reviews should not only review previous data systematically, they should systematically evaluate the quality of those data (Jüni, Altman, and Egger 2001). To be sure, the best of all systems would be one that prized "less research, better research, and research done for the right reasons" (Altman 1994: 284). Alas, the reward structure for biomedical scientists, at least for those in academia, tends to emphasize quantity over quality, with a number of undesirable results (recall the "publication fetishists" from Chapter 1). Part of the problem faced by those who seek to synthesize research is that they are faced with a great deal of slop, chaff and pseudo-data, all tarted up to beguile and deceive, and as often as not utterly nugatory.

This reward structure has also contributed to what is perhaps the best-known scientific corpus corruptor – publication bias. This is the phenomenon by which, firstly, journal editors and referees over-select submissions that report clearly positive (or sometimes clearly negative) results, or are supported by outside funding, and, secondly, investigators themselves withhold and otherwise under-submit reports of projects that do not evince dramatic results (i.e., apparently because they know of publication bias and so believe that their work would not receive a fair appraisal, thus turning publication bias into a kind of self-fulfilling prophecy). This is called the "file drawer problem."

So, not only are individual reports flawed, the very fabric of scientific communication is sullied by social forces beyond the control of the systematic reviewer. The good news/bad news story here is that almost immediately upon the discovery of the publication bias' effect on meta-analyses, the research community moved to identify and study it, and reduce its influence (e.g., Dickersin et al. 1987; Newcombe 1987; Chalmers 1990; Dickersin

1990; Easterbrook et al. 1991; Dickersin, Min, and Meinert 1992; Dickersin and Min 1993a, b; Sutton et al. 2000; Sterne, Egger, and Smith 2001). We have further discovered that the corpus is bloated by redundancy: In one noteworthy case involving a major quality-of-life issue, "a quarter of all relevant published reports are duplicates" (Tramèr et al. 1997: 1088). This general redundancy is caused (motivated?) by academic arm-waving, commercial influence, sponsorship pressures, and – despite the earnest and vehement protests of investigators who avow with fist pumping and carotid bulging – outright conflicts of interest and commitment.[14]

One obvious way to address these problems – well it is obvious nowadays – is to establish comprehensive, high-quality repositories of data, independent of their publication status. This, too, was proposed early on in the current meta-analysis period (Simes 1986; Chalmers, Frank, and Reitman 1990) and has continued (Horton and Smith 1999; Smith and Horton 1999). Recall also that Archie Cochrane's goal of making available a "critical summary, by specialty or subspecialty, adapted periodically, of all relevant randomized controlled trials" makes no reference to the trials' publication status. The brute fact of publication bias ends up providing added impetus to the realization of Cochrane's dream in the Cochrane Collaboration (Chalmers, Dickersin, and Chalmers 1992; Warren and Mosteller 1993; Bero and Rennie 1995). One upshot – The Cochrane Controlled Trials Register – "is a bibliographic database of controlled trials identified by contributors to the Cochrane Collaboration and others, as part of an international effort to systematically search the world's health care journals and other sources of information, and create an unbiased source of data for systematic reviews" (Cochrane Collaboration 2001).

But we should slow down a little. As every scientist, scholar, or investigator who has had a paper rejected by a journal knows, biomedical journal editors are: (1) morons, (2) fascist morons, (3) mutant fascist morons, or (4) necrophiliac mutant fascist morons. This belief is held with a certainty not easily weakened by acknowledgment that the proffered article might actually be reporting on a study that was poorly designed, sloppily executed, or statistically fallacious. (When papers are accepted for publication, this is sometimes regarded as evidence of the editor's insight, genius, compassion, and good looks.) That is, for all that is wrong with peer review, it is, at its best, a generally fair attempt to introduce some measure of quality and rigor into the scientific publication process. It might be, that is, that the paper was rejected by the journal because it was not good enough to publish (Erwin

1984). It follows from this that a registry that included all such unpublished reports, in the interest of comprehensiveness and to avoid the problem of publication bias, might be a registry populated by (some? many?) reports of low quality.

This points us in an interesting direction, namely that systematic reviews, done well, *become* a kind of peer review. In fact, the notion that clinical trial quality should itself be the subject of objective evaluation has been the source of extraordinary research and intense debate. Indeed, one might suggest that a systematic review simply must include an assessment of the quality of the studies it builds on. According to the *Cochrane Reviewers' Handbook*:

Quality assessment of individual studies that are summarised in systematic reviews is necessary to limit bias in conducting the systematic review, gain insight into potential comparisons, and guide interpretation of findings. Factors that warrant assessment are those related to applicability of findings, validity of individual studies, and certain design characteristics that affect interpretation of results. Applicability, which is also called external validity or generalisability by some, is related to the definition of the key components of well-formulated questions . . . Specifically, whether a review's findings are applicable to a particular population, intervention strategy or outcome is dependent upon the studies selected for review, and on how the people, interventions and outcomes of interest were defined by these studies and the reviewers.

Interpretation of results is dependent upon the validity of the included studies and other characteristics. For example, a review may summarise twenty valid trials that evaluate the effects of anti-ischemic agents on symptoms of chest pain in adults with prior myocardial infarction. However, the trials may examine different preparations and doses of anti-ischemic agents and may have varying durations. These latter issues would affect interpretation though they may not be directly relevant to the internal validity of the trials. (Clarke and Oxman 2001: section 6)

Quality can be assessed more or less formally, and each direction has its virtues and drawbacks. What seems to be clear is that the creation and evaluation of scales and checklists for quality assessment, as for instance in the important work by Alex Jadad, David Moher, and their colleagues (e.g., Moher et al. 1995; Jadad et al. 1996; Moher, Jadad, and Tugwell 1996), is a necessary and positive development – even as it elicits its own critical literature (Clark et al. 1999; Jüni et al. 1999) on the "quality of assessing quality" (Berlin and Rennie 1999: 1084).

Now, it would be splendid if studies were reported in such a way as to make facile these quality assessments. In fact, studies are often reported with great variability, low quality and inconsistent data. This has led a consortium of scientists and editors to develop protocols to standardize and improve the quality of reports of randomized controlled trials. The "Consolidated Standards of Reporting Trials" (CONSORT) statement, drafted in 1996 (Begg et al. 1996) and revised in 2001 (Altman et al. 2001; a number of cognate reports were published in other British and North American medical journals) contains a checklist of items to include when reporting a trial, a template to demonstrate flow of patients through a trial, and other guidelines for data sharing. And, of course, such standards require evaluation before we should attach too much weight to them; one such evaluation concluded that use of the CONSORT checklist "may be associated with improving the quality of reports of RCTs [randomized controlled trials]. Higher-quality reports are likely to improve RCT interpretation, minimize biased conclusions, and ultimately facilitate decision making about treatment effectiveness" (Moher, Jones, and Lepage 2001: 1995).

Explanatory uncertainty and regress

There is no stopping us now. If we are going to systematize the reporting of trials – and we ought – then why not systematize the reporting of systematic reviews of trials? This is the goal of the Quality of Reporting of Meta-Analyses (QUOROM) statement, which addresses issues related to searching for studies, to include: selection of those studies, validity assessment, data abstraction, study characteristics, data synthesis, etc. (Moher et al. 1999).

One should be forgiven the impression that the house of biomedical science is leaking like a sieve, and that there is an urgent and ongoing effort to patch the leaks as soon as they are noticed.

There is, of course, no alternative. The insight that gave rise to evidence-based practice is a strict, even cruel, mistress. It is not out of sentiment or courtesy that we insist that clinical decisions be based on the best available evidence; it is not because the boffins of academia have conspired to make miserable the lives of community clinicians; and it is not because someone has surreptitiously cornered the market in medical epistemology and is in line to make a few bucks or quid in the process. Science and morality jointly demand that evidence be integrated into clinical practice because there is good reason to believe that when it is, people live better, happier, healthier, and longer. Any clinician who does not like this, or who has a fundamental disagreement with the idea, has made a grave error in his or her career choice.

But that tautology notwithstanding, we may also be forgiven the fear, the hesitancy, and the *scientific* uncertainty that arises from legitimate disagreements within the evidence-based edifice. Put differently, evidence-based practice should guide the clinician, but it cannot – it just cannot – give us the kind of conceptual closure so many clinicians either crave or demand. If anything, it sometimes seems to be taking back as much as it gives. The conceptual hurdle we face is formed by a series of potential regresses:

- Conduct a trial → evaluate the quality of the trial → evaluate the quality of the instrument used to evaluate the quality of the trial . . .
- Conduct a systematic review → evaluate the quality of the review (including the quality of the instrument used to evaluate the quality of the trials used in the review) → evaluate the quality of the instrument used to evaluate the quality of the review . . .
- Construct a practice guideline that embodies reviews (evaluated for quality) based on trials (evaluated for quality) → evaluate the quality of the guideline (including the quality of the instrument used to evaluate the quality of the trials and the quality of the instrument used to evaluate the quality of the trials used in the review) → evaluate the quality of the instrument used to evaluate the quality of the guideline . . .

Each step in each task is plausibly required to reduce bias, avoid error, and maintain quality. We will need a principled way of addressing these regresses – a stance to take toward them – and this will come later (in Chapters 5 and 7), when we weave together the threads now being colored by uncertainty, fallibility, and conceptual and pedagogic diligence. We will not, however, eliminate uncertainty. Indeed, we cannot eliminate it, at least not in many cases (often perhaps the most difficult ones). The increasing demands of evidence-based practice will be best seen not as demands to eliminate uncertainty but, rather, tools to cope with it. These tools are conceptual and they are moral.

Still, regresses are unhappy things, and I should give a sense of how we might set them aside. I will do this by listening to the voices of those who are prepared to endure uncertainty by insisting on more science.

Keep in mind the reasons for all these secondary reviews, evaluations, and assessments in the first place. The reasons I am thinking of include complexity, scientific progress, and variable quality. By "complexity" I just mean that the systems we are studying and trying to treat have numerous moving parts and it is sometimes or often difficult to tell how they all fit together: "Biological and social systems are inherently complex, so it is hardly surprising that few if any human illnesses can be said to have a single 'cause' or 'cure'" (Wilson and Holt 2001: 685; cf. Plsek and Greenhalgh 2001). It is therefore to be expected that we will not get it right the first time.

"Scientific progress" means simply that we know more than we used to, and our tools for finding things out are better than they used to be. Our ability to make medical observations, conduct clinical trials, and perform reviews of trials is improving all the time. Some of the frustration we experience at seeing new layers of inquiry and evaluation might just as well be excitement fired by recognition of the improvement in our ability to see what makes the world work.

"Variable quality" is that part of the biomedical inquiry that we could have done a better job on the first time around: Poorly designed trials, sloppy statistics, social pressures to force-feed and fatten up the scientific corpus like a goose whose liver we intend to have our way with – these are all motivators and causes of efforts to do better next time. If we were able to do it all over again, we would spend more time teaching medical, pharmacology, physiology, nursing, psychology, epidemiology, psychology and other students how to do research properly, we would insist on scientists and clinicians being rewarded by means other than those that celebrate the thickness of a CV or the decimal points from external funding, and we would ensure adequate and international support for, and access to, the very best of our efforts.[15]

Furthermore, what is troubling us about regressive aspects of attempts to improve the quality of the evidence in evidence-based medicine is actually not unique in biomedicine. In any science, one who wants to drill down as far as possible in search of foundations for belief will always find more and more opportunities to postpone the denouement. It is only when the upshot of our experiments can have so immediate and direct a human consequence that we so often want and need to double-check our work. We might also in the process just learn more about our science. Here are three examples:

(1) There are several ways to conduct a meta-analysis. One might, for instance, do a meta-analysis based on data from published studies, or one might use individual patient data. Are there grounds to prefer either method over the other? Are those grounds general or do they apply only for certain kinds of reviews? The only way to answer these and other questions in applied statistics is to conduct a comparison, a

sort of meta-meta-analysis. As it develops, there is said to be "excellent quantitative agreement between the summary effect estimates" of both methods, but each has other advantages (Steinberg et al. 1997: 917). While we might want to compare future studies that likewise themselves compared published and patient data – and thereby risk another regress – we more rationally will decide whether to conduct a study of studies depending on what kinds of questions we want to answer. That there is another layer to peel away is not a fault of method, but a feature of the structure of biomedical reality.[16]

(2) There is an urgent need to compare systematic reviews in the published literature with those prepared by scientific societies and by entities such as the Cochrane Collaboration or the US Agency for Healthcare Research and Quality (AHRQ).[17] Reasons for this include determination of which reviews are updated most regularly and therefore are of greatest clinical utility, and to guide those who would conduct future human subjects research or, as part of institutional review boards or research ethics committees, *oversee* that research. This question – against what scientific background is it permissible to allow subjects to be exposed to risk? – is among the most interesting and difficult in all research (and we will return to it in Chapter 7). The answer will depend in part on the confidence we place on the best syntheses of our knowledge in a domain. If our confidence is high that a clinical research question has been adequately addressed, then it becomes unethical to allow humans to be exposed to risk as part of efforts to continue to address that same question. Because of comparisons of the sort being discussed here, we can say with warrant that traditionally published systematic reviews lack some of the methodological rigor of, and are not updated as frequently as, say, reviews by the Cochrane Collaboration (e.g., Jadad et al. 1998; Jadad et al. 2000; Olsen et al. 2001); indeed, all aspects of review repositories should be reviewed (Petticrew et al. 1999) along with practice guidelines (Hayward et al. 1995; Wilson et al. 1995; Weingarten 1997).

(3) The network of reviews of reviews, or meta-reviews if you like, is contributing to an extraordinarily important debate about study design. Should clinical trials be randomized? Why? It turns out that there is some evidence from systematic reviews to suggest that randomization might *not* be needed to ensure the quality of a clinical trial (Benson and Hartz 2000; Concato, Shah and Horowitz 2000; Ioannidis et al. 2001).

But the consequences of eliminating this traditional methodological buffer against bias might be too great to permit (Pocock and Elbourne 2000). This debate is fantastically interesting and important. It is also unsettled; this is a state of affairs in science that is best addressed by more science.

The practical utility of systematic reviews

Meta-analysis and other systematic reviews have been subjected to withering criticism, some of it based on concerns, such as publication bias, already noted here, and generally based on misgivings about clinical inferences from indirect evidence. Perhaps poetic license will permit the concatenation of some favorite epithets:

> Meta-analysis "offers the Holy Grail of attaining statistically stable estimates for effects of low magnitude" (Shapiro 1994: 771) because it is "statistical alchemy" (Feinstein 1995: 71) that is "devoid of original thought" (Rosendaal 1994: 1325) and an exemplar of "mega-silliness" (Eysenck 1978).

Strong opinions can help scientific disputes retain their interest. What we need now, given that systematic reviews and research synthesis have become fixtures in the epistemological firmament, is clearer focus of their domains of greatest applicability, their limits, their most appropriate contexts of use. The sense I have so far tried to instill is that the science of research synthesis is itself in ferment, and rationality permits neither slavish devotion nor skeptical dismissal. There is no arguing with someone who insists that medical decisions should be based on the "best available evidence." The arguing takes place over what constitutes this evidence, how one knows when one has it (and not some other thing) and, failing that, where to find it. That is where the best and most important debates occur, and that is the uncertainty that shapes our ethical tension.

One way to make this explicit is to look at a few challenges to (or concerns about) the practical utility of systematic reviews. It is a way of broadening still further the uncertainty that must accompany certain clinical decisions.

Consider first that the best evidence applies to populations that are the best studied, and it is well known that some populations, including women, minorities, children, and elders, are under-represented in study cohorts. While this is changing, it is nevertheless unclear how or to what extent to apply the syntheses of studies "performed on a homogeneous study population [and which] exclude clinically complex cases for the sake of internal validity" (Knottnerus and Dinant 1997: 1109; cf. Feinstein and Horwitz 1997). Indeed, systematic reviews have long been known to suffer from the "heterogeneity problem," or what has been called the problem of "apples and oranges" and which has always been acknowledged by proponents (Hunter and Schmidt 1990; Chalmers 1991; Thompson 1994). Heterogeneous data can be integrated (Mulrow, Langhorne, and Grimshaw 1997); indeed, it might even be that the process of heterogeneity identification can be computerized (Costa-Bouzas et al. 2001), but it will be some time before we can, for many subgroups, identify the clinical upshots of this integration.

Consider next that it is not just population subgroups but entire populations that might be overlooked by the best evidence. Listen to the view from Fiji:

Evidence-based medicine – where the term is used in the more formal sense – has unfortunately only limited applicability in Fiji and the less-developed world in general. The cost of generating and using the best possible epidemiological evidence is high, and the external validity of high-quality evidence in the Fijian setting is often questionable. Key issues in medical care here must continue to be researched, with the highest possible methodological standards, but in some instances these standards may need to be set lower than in more developed countries. (Lowe 2000: 1107)

It is a (so far) unremarked irony that epidemiology, the science that in many ways has taught us the most about systematic health science (which, as it turns out, evolved in and is firstly applicable to comparatively wealthy and already well-studied populations), is also the science that has taught us that what developing countries mostly need is not magnetic resonance imaging, organ transplantation, or sophisticated statistical resources, but clean water and adequate waste disposal services.

Generally, meta-analysis and other systematic reviews need to be evaluated in terms of how broad a piece of the practice and policy spectrum they should occupy, how many minutes of arc they should subsume. Some statisticians have argued for an extremely limited role for meta-analysis, albeit largely as a result of errors attributed to the method and not because of conceptual concerns related to its meta-evidentiary status. The statistician John Bailar, for instance, would grant meta-analysis "a potentially useful role in carefully selected situations where the primary literature is of good quality, heterogeneity in response to treatment of the tested population is small and well understood, interest centers on estimation of a specific, critical parameter of outcome, and the meta-analyst is deeply expert in the subject matter" (Bailar 1995).

This is a small house and one with very tight security. Advocates of the new evidence find it oppressive. Pity the world of illness, disability and death, when it must choose between competing statisticians! But the balance that needs to be struck is one with which we now should be familiar. We want the fulcrum of medical and public health decision making to be placed in such a way as to minimize bad things and maximize good ones. This is exactly what we always wanted, of course, and always in contexts similarly shaped by uncertainty. Now, though, with more science on the balance, we have come to expect a great deal.

How to read the "how to read the medical literature" literature

Meta-evidence had engendered its own meta-commentary. If clinicians are to make the most of the new evidence – and if it is ethically blameworthy if they do not – then editors and educators are similarly duty bound to create some kind of evidence-based re-education system. They have done their duty, more or less. Mainly, they have produced a body of work that attempts to show clinicians how to learn from the contemporary literature, a pedagogic task that until recently was ignored in most medical education and continuing education.

The *Journal of the American Medical Association*, for instance, produced a series of high-quality articles comprising "Users' Guides to the Medical Literature," covering topics ranging from "How to use articles about clinical decision rules" to "How to use an article measuring the effect of an intervention on surrogate end points;" the series is redacted into a volume billed as being both "detailed" and "clinically friendly" (Guyatt and Rennie 2001). The *British Medical Journal* regularly distills for readers its articles' evidence-based take-home points and like *JAMA* has seen its publisher issue a volume devoted to the topic (Greenhalgh 2000).

This is generally the literature of advocacy. It seeks to win over skeptics. It succeeds in those cases in which clinicians come to accept the philosophical underpinnings of the evidence-based medicine movement and incorporate (at least some of) its principles into their practices. And to the extent that evidence-based practice improves patient care, there is an ethical imperative to undertake such an incorporation. As a literature of advocacy, though, its stance is Oslerian – recall the "simple" and "self-evident" advice that "To get an accurate knowledge of any disease it is necessary to study a large series of cases and to go into all the particulars." Should the busy clinician trying to parse an interminable heap of medical scholarship take this stance, or the stance of those who, at least in terms of meta-analysis, caution against too facile a reading of the latest synthesis?

Or maybe there is no great difference here at all; maybe we are selling Osler short. He is, after all, calling for the study of a "large series of cases" in all their particulars – we might rather regard this as anticipating precisely the kind of systematic review and guideline creation that form the foundation of a solid evidence-based practice. The only difference is that Osler is not (yet) a partisan in a movement, but an observer who sees the simple and self-evident truth that we learn from our probings of the world, and that rational care is at some unspecified level based on publicly observable data that we render into evidence.

The "how to read the medical literature" literature tends not to highlight the actual and potential shortcomings of systematic science. Rather, it battles against apparently wide ignorance of some core concepts of randomized controlled trials and evidence-based practice. For instance, while most general practitioners in a UK questionnaire survey reported using evidence-based summaries in their practices, precious few understood or were able to explain the simple, crucial, and widely ignored concept of number needed to treat (McColl et al. 1998, cited by Sackett et al. 2000; cf. McQuay and Moore 1997), or the number of patients one needs to treat to prevent an additional bad outcome.[18] This matters a great deal, especially regarding informed consent, because patients will make different decisions depending on whether information emphasizes relative or absolute risk reduction, number needed to treat, or personal probability of benefit (Misselbrook and Armstrong 2001, cited in a very important defense of better public understanding of clinical trials: Horton 2001a).

In this respect, the "how to read the literature" literature provides, for many clinicians, that part of the science education they never had. Integrated into clinical education, systematic reviews can help provide a useful and indeed powerful introduction to core concepts of systematic clinical research (Badgett, O'Keefe, and Henderson 1997). Indeed, this "how to" literature would benefit by sharing more widely with ordinary clinicians some of the straightforward and intuitively powerful insights that are used in the how-to literature for those who are already conducting the reviews. Keeping in mind our discussions about causation and confirmation, consider how someone conducting a systematic review of clinical trials might borrow from Austin Bradford Hill's famous criteria (Hill 1971: 312ff.) for evaluating causal inferences:

- How good is the quality of the included trials?
- How large and significant are the observed effects?
- How consistent are the effects across trials?
- Is there a clear dose–response relationship?
- Is there indirect evidence that supports the inference?
- Have other plausible competing explanations of the observed effects (e.g., bias or co-intervention) been ruled out? (Clarke and Oxman 2001: 84, cf. Oxman in press)

In other words, ordinary clinicians who are suspicious of systematic medical science might be well served by reassurance that the meta-evidence they suspect, fear or scorn is in fact capable of identifying causal relations.

Like any scientific literature, however, the "how to read the medical literature" corpus will strengthen its own credibility with a robust and frank incorporation of its greatest weaknesses as well as its greatest strengths. And, like all literatures whose authors care about the results (even if they have a good reason for caring), we should regard advocacy as raising the possibility of a sort of conceptual conflict of interest: It does not mean they are not to be believed, only that evidence and evidence alone is required to build and shape belief. That we must almost always take a grain of salt with our evidence, and especially our new meta-evidence, is a mark of prudence and caution, not skepticism or disdain.

NOTES

1 Cited in Frank (1949) and Clark (1971).
2 The idea that scientific theories are underdetermined by evidence was one of the most important issues in twentieth century philosophy of science. Sometimes called the "Quine–Duhem (or Duhem–Quine) thesis," the contention is that scientific theories are underdetermined by physical evidence such that no evidence could ever settle a dispute over which theory to accept – could not decide the question of which theory was superior – in part because the theories could be modified to take into account any evidence (Quine 1953; Duhem 1962). We are concerned here not with

scientific theories but with diagnoses, treatment efficacy, prognoses, etc., or what we can call "clinical theories," but similar issues can apply.

3 An interesting question in the philosophy of science relates to whether confirmation is differential, that is whether evidence that confirms a theory must also be evidence against a competing theory, or whether evidence disconfirming a theory becomes evidence that confirms a competitor. Edward Erwin and Harvey Siegel contend that confirmation is differential for scientific theories (Erwin and Siegel 1989). It is not clear, however, whether confirmation of a diagnosis by some bit of clinical evidence thereby is simultaneously evidence against competing diagnoses. It would seem strange if this were so, and at any rate it would go against the very idea of using differential diagnoses in education and, especially, in clinical practice.

4 The history of clinical trials is nicely addressed by a website, "Controlled trials from history," created by the Royal College of Physicians of Edinburgh (available at http://www.rcpe.ac.uk/controlled_trials/index.html2001) and by the *British Medical Journal* in a special issue, "The randomised controlled trial at 50" (October 31, 1998, available at http://www.bmj.com/content/vol317/issue7167/).

5 The same confusion, from a patient's perspective: ". . . following the recent deaths . . . in government-sponsored clinical trials at two major American universities, some have questioned why, in the era of transgenic mice and computer modeling of molecules, we still experiment on people. As one patient recently asked, 'Why don't they just give us the good stuff?'" (Shaywitz and Ausiello 2001).

6 We must say "usually" here because while, for our purposes, we are thinking about people or their parts (sometimes very small parts), scientists often perform experiments on, or involving, entities which may not be objects, at least in the ordinary use of the term and at the time of the experiment. The equivalence of matter and energy does not absolve us from thinking of various forms of radiation, for instance, as distinct from most physical objects.

7 We need to hedge by implying that there might be *some* reason to doubt external causation in order to accommodate (and hence set aside) counterexamples that appeal to dreams, hallucinations, ciguatera poisoning, etc.

8 Specifically – and note the causal chain – "Aspirin causes irreversible inhibition of platelet cyclo-oxygenase, thereby preventing formation of thromboxane A_2, a platelet aggregant and potent vasoconstrictor" (Cairns et al. 1998, citing Stein and Fuster 1992). Uncertainty arises, as we shall see, from the simple fact that this straightforward mechanism either does not always occur or, if it does occur, does not always work to reduce mortality.

9 The ellipsis may be required to capture the fact that we should probably regard "reduce mortality" not as a distinct event but as a series of numerous events with the feature "not die," or, more precisely, a series of events in which platelet aggregation has been inhibited such that had this inhibition not occurred the patient would (more likely) have died. To be sure, the question as to whether this reduces mortality in a

specific case is a question that cannot be answered in the absence of more information about the patient.

10 Indeed, it might be based on any number of guidelines, recommendations, and commentaries that rely on either or both other sources of evidence (e.g., Ryan et al. 1999; Spinler et al. 2001). Here we are conspicuously avoiding other considerations which complicate the issue, but which any competent clinician would need to take into account. These include consideration of the likelihood that some patients will have an adverse reaction to aspirin; which alternative therapies would be most appropriate; etc.

11 A comprehensive meta-analysis/systematic review literature has emerged, providing evidence for the utility, resilience, and intellectual excitement of such methods: Hedges and Olkin 1985; Wachter and Straf 1990; Cook et al. 1992; Cooper and Hedges 1994; Colditz, Glasziou, and Irwig 2001. Systematic reviews have even fallen foul of various – and sometimes unfair – myths and misconceptions (Petticrew 2001), which perhaps have impeded acceptance of evidence-based medicine by some clinicians.

12 While this might be grist for another project, biomedical researchers have generally been less than rigorous in their use of the various terms for aggregating the results of disparate studies. For our purposes, and given that the same conceptual, methodological, and ethical issues are in play for all such aggregations, not much hangs on this question here. This is not to say it is not an important question, and a noteworthy exception to terminological laxity emerged from what was called the "Potsdam consultation":

Systematic review = overview = the application of scientific strategies that limit bias to the systematic assembly, critical appraisal, and synthesis of all relevant studies on a specific topic. Meta-analysis = quantitative overview = a systematic review that employs statistical methods to combine and summarize the results of several studies. (Cook, Sackett, and Spitzer 1995: 167)

13 An omitted footnote points to a touchstone article by the Evidence-based Medicine Working Group (1992), which announces that "A new paradigm for medical practice is emerging. Evidence-based medicine de-emphasizes intuition, unsystematic clinical experience, and pathophysiological rationale as sufficient grounds for clinical decision making and stresses the examination of evidence from clinical research" (p. 2420).

14 This point is emphatically intended to be general and not to apply to any *particular or specific* (set) of publications.

15 The idea that some of the best of our medical and public health excellence is hidden behind pay-per-view websites – structured so as to prevent unauthorized access (as if a physician looking for a trial result were somehow like an adolescent scouting about for free smut!) – is as sure a sign of barbarism as if we intentionally set about

trying to kill or torture the people whose lives will be lost or suffering increased because of inaccessible scientific data.

16 Similar points could be made regarding those meta-analyses that use fixed effects and those that use random effects (see Villar et al. 2001).

17 The AHRQ's important Evidence-based Practice Centers "review all relevant scientific literature on assigned clinical care topics and produce evidence reports and technology assessments, conduct research on methodologies and the effectiveness of their implementation, and participate in technical assistance activities. Public and private sector organizations may use the reports and assessments as the basis for their own clinical guidelines and other quality improvement activities" (Agency for Healthcare Research and Quality 2001a). The agency's National Guideline Clearinghouse provides a free, online "mechanism for obtaining objective, detailed information on clinical practice guidelines and to further their dissemination, implementation and use" (Agency for Healthcare Research and Quality 2001b).

18 Consider the following from the glossary of the National Health Service's Centre for Evidence-Based Medicine, a very useful website:

The Number Needed to Treat (NNT) is the number of patients you need to treat to prevent one additional bad outcome (death, stroke, etc.). For example, if a drug has an NNT of 5, it means you have to treat 5 people with the drug to prevent one additional bad outcome. . . . To calculate the NNT, you need to know the Absolute Risk Reduction (ARR); the NNT is the inverse of the ARR:

NNT = 1/ARR

Where ARR = CER (Control Event Rate) − EER (Experimental Event Rate) and "event rate" is the proportion of patients in a group in whom an event is observed. Thus, if out of 100 patients, the event is observed in 27, the event rate is 0.27. Control Event Rate (CER) and Experimental Event Rate (EER) are used to refer to this in control and experimental groups of patients respectively (National Health Service 2001).

So, for instance, recalling the ISIS-2 study cited earlier, it develops that the NNT to prevent death with aspirin therapy after an acute myocardial infarction is greater than 20. NNTs tend to put research into perspective and make clear (to clinicians and lay people) that breathless news media reports are often misleading. Note also in this regard the consistent confusion of absolute and relative risk reduction. It would be interesting to study the effect of evidence-based practice on patient adherence to treatment or drug regimens; one might hypothesize that if they had a truer or more accurate picture of the effects of an intervention, patients would not bother as much to follow their clinicians' recommendations or treatment plan.

4

Human subjects, the Internet, databases, and data mining

Even the wisest of doctors are relying on scientific truths the errors of which will be recognized within a few years time.[1]   Proust

The randomized, double-blind, placebo-controlled trial, about a half-century old, is reckoned to be the gold standard for acquiring evidence in medicine. Indeed, the randomized controlled trial (RCT) is the engine of evidence-based practice. But such trials are often either inapplicable or impossible, or they are in keen need of volunteers – both situations in which the Internet has been enlisted. Indeed, the use of computers and related tools to seek, gather, store, analyze, and share personal health information poses interesting and difficult ethical challenges, especially given advances in knowledge discovery in databases, in terms of the requirements of informed or valid consent, and facing the increased evidentiary burdens of contemporary practice. The stakes can be very high, indeed, when computers, consent, and confidentiality intersect as scientists try to develop early warning systems for bioterrorism.

Computers and consent

It is a common and unhappy misconception among health professionals that bioethics is a source of problems, controversies, and, worse, dilemmas rather than a source of solutions. In fact, bioethics has solved far more problems than it has raised, and it is only a kind of dilemma fetishism that has obscured this achievement: We savor and trade tales of intractability and discord like numismatists, philatelists, or children with Japanese game cards – the greater the error or conflict, the more valuable or reliable the currency, somehow.

The best example of success or progress in bioethics is that of the development of the concept of informed or valid consent. Foreshadowed by the philosophy of Immanuel Kant, shaped in the crucible of Nuremberg, and fumbled after in postwar courtrooms, valid consent now enjoys interdisciplinary support, international credibility, and the sort of conceptual traction that gives an idea practical utility in the boardroom and at the bedside. Valid consent has solved numerous problems in clinical practice and human subjects research. The law and the ethics are congruent. It is intuitively straightforward and easily accessible to lay people.

It is, in short, one of the greatest examples of conceptual problem solving in the history of human inquiry.

That said, the value of the concept of valid consent must be tested, validated, or evaluated anew in a dizzying variety of contexts if it is not to be relegated to the museum of formerly useful notions. The core components of valid consent – adequate information, voluntariness, and capacity or competence – may be subject to challenges and critiques we have not thought of yet, and they are often taken for granted. Put differently: For all its success, the concept of valid consent should inspire us to curiosity and vigilance, not complacency. This is because the sciences of clinical practice and human subjects research are themselves evolving rapidly and it is in these sciences that we expect valid consent to do the heavy lifting.

The new contexts or domains in which valid consent must be challenged include genetics, health services research, and the Internet (and other information technologies). The last of these offers a superb opportunity to study consent because it is rapidly subsuming the others or including them among its subclasses, and we can further appeal to a new and growing interest in ethical issues in health informatics.[2]

The intersection of "computing" and "consent" therefore offers us an exciting series of challenges, as well as a variety of venues for further research. Indeed, at a number of places in the discussion that follows, we will be wishing that more of that research had already been done. For instance, do on-line clinical trial listings affirm or subvert the requirements of valid consent? Can the Internet be used to obtain consent? Can computers be used to manage data so as to reduce the need for consent for research on databases? These are, in part, empirical questions – questions whose answers will determine whether the foundation of valid consent will support larger and more varied structures.

In what follows I address use of the Internet and World Wide Web for recruiting subjects and as a target of research itself. The requirements of valid consent will be seen to provide a solid foundation for ethically optimizing research, although information technology also will be seen to raise special challenges for the consent process. I'll also examine the use of databases to store information and as places to conduct further research on that information through a process or technique known as "data mining." Again, the requirements of valid consent will be seen generally to provide a solid foundation for ethically optimizing this research, although information technology consistently is seen to raise a broad variety of interesting challenges.

On-line research and research on-line

Recruiting subjects

We have, in an extraordinarily short time, transformed the way in which patients learn about clinical trials. Indeed, the very notion of patients *learning about* clinical trials – implying some educational or other benefit – is novel. Traditionally, it was only through one's physician that one heard of a drug or device experiment. Generally speaking, a patient would be included as a subject only if:

- the trial was for an intervention for a non-serious malady, so if the experiment failed there was little harm done; or
- there was no standard treatment for a serious malady, so, while there might be the risk of (nontrivial) harm, it could be a risk worth taking; or
- there was a treatment for a serious malady, but it had failed.

Now, though, patients and patient groups are increasingly insisting on information about drug and device experiments. Given the success of the biomedical research enterprise, it is not surprising that patients would insist on "ready access to information about clinical research studies so that they might be more fully informed about a range of potential treatment options, particularly for very serious diseases" (McCray and Ide 2000: 313).

In response to such demands, the US Congress – through the Food and Drug Administration's Modernization Act – ordered that information about clinical trials be made more easily available through Web-based technology.[3] The result: In early 2000, the National Institutes of Health, through the National Library of Medicine, launched "ClinicalTrials.gov," an on-line resource to provide "a single place you can go where the most important information, we hope, will be available to everybody" (Associated Press 2000). Patients, family members, and others (with Internet access) can browse the 5000 listed studies. Most of the studies are NIH-sponsored, but experiments from other sponsors, including the pharmaceutical industry, are to be included. Additionally, many cancer, AIDS, and other specific research units, universities, and other entities maintain on-line lists of trials.

This is all to the good, so far: Patients and family members seeking one-stop shopping in their searches for new or better treatments for serious maladies. Given that the government sponsors as much research as it does, it might even be blameworthy if it did not make something like ClinicalTrials.gov available. But here we must be very careful, and make two crucial distinctions:

(1) Lists vs. solicitations. The first distinction is between (1) an on-line *list* of studies, and (2) a mechanism for *recruiting* subjects into those studies. The difference between informing and recruiting can be quite subtle, but the upshot is always significant. The point at which one begins to recruit subjects normally should trigger a broad ensemble of ethical and legal protections. Most significant among these is review by an institutional review board (IRB) or research ethics committee. Under US law, IRBs must review all advertisements and other means of recruiting subjects.

(2) Experiments vs. treatments. Clinical trials are undertaken because there is insufficient warrant to regard a particular drug or device as safe and effective; that is, we often do experiments to find out whether a particular drug or device is safe and effective, or to test the relative effectiveness of two or more drugs for which there are already data on safety and effectiveness. We must therefore take great pains to distinguish between (1) *experiments* or tests, studies, or trials and (2) *treatments*, or the drugs and devices for which we do have sufficient warrant to regard as safe and effective.

Let us be clear about why (aside from mere curiosity) a patient might seek out an academic, corporate, disease center, government, or other on-line list of clinical trials: Either there is no standard treatment for his or her malady, or the standard treatment has failed – two of the three reasons why patients would traditionally seek and/or receive a physician's referral to a trial. The concern we now face is that (1) on-line listings will have the effect of *recruiting* subjects, and (2) the subjects will regard the experimental interventions as *treatments*. In other words, having made two important distinctions, we have reason to fear that sick people will find themselves on the most problematic side of both of them.

Patients and subjects labor under what is called the "therapeutic misconception" (Appelbaum et al. 1987), when they believe with inadequate reason that an experimental intervention or process will work. Consider now the following language from one university-based website:

Clinical research trials are very rewarding for both the patient and the physician. The patient may benefit from new treatment options and help future cancer patients in their fight against this disease. [This site] strongly recommends patients discuss any clinical research trials for which they may be eligible with their oncologist.

And this from ClinicalTrials.gov (answering the question "why volunteer?"):

By taking part in a clinical trial, you can try a new treatment that may or may not be better than those already available. You can also contribute to better understanding of how the treatment works in people of different ethnic backgrounds and genders.

And this from a Department of Veterans Affairs' description of a collaboration with the National Cancer Institute:

People take part in clinical trials for many reasons. They may hope for a cure of disease, a longer time to live, a way to feel better, or a way to prevent cancer. Patients usually hope the trial will benefit them personally. Often, they also want to contribute to a research effort that may help others. There are drawbacks to consider, including possible side effects and time commitment. Some studies may require treatment schedules that conflict with work and family responsibilities. Learn as much as you can about a study before you decide to participate. (Department of Veterans Affairs 2001)

And this heading from one corporate clinical trial matchmaking service: "Join a clinical study"– as if it were a social club or soccer team.

It does not require hyperbolic skepticism to fear that the message being communicated is not one of caution but of opportunity, and, hence, that the therapeutic misconception is being encouraged or reinforced instead of being reduced or eliminated. Here is one way to express this concern:

Before an intervention is demonstrated to be effective it is not even clear that we want to call it a treatment; we reserve that term for drugs, devices and procedures we have reason to believe will work. Suggesting otherwise is to go beyond the evidence and perhaps even to engender false hope. . . . The question of how potential trial subjects are best informed of the availability of trials is complicated by the language used to describe the research enterprise. Are patients on trials "subjects" or "participants"? Are they "eligible" (as if for a contest) or do they meet "inclusion criteria"? Do they receive a "treatment" or are they involved in an "experiment"? To describe a study as if it were likely to produce a benefit is unacceptable. (Goodman 2000)

But it remains to be seen how great an effect the medium – the World Wide Web – has on these issues. Does it engender distrust between physicians and patients, especially in the case of a desperate patient inferring a likely benefit from an inadequately studied intervention? Does it engender false hope? How many patients will mistakenly infer some, even minimal, level of official or academic imprimatur or endorsement? Do they suffer from the "computational fallacy" or "the view that what comes out of a computer is somehow more valid, accurate, or reliable" than anything a human can or might produce? (Goodman 1998d)

Actually, matters may be complicated somewhat by pre-existing failures of public trust. *Lancet* editor Richard Horton lists five propositions about clinical trials, "all of which undermine their scientific and ethical validity" (Horton 2001a: 593): Trials are deceitful, disputable, unbelievable, unhelpful, and shameful. These perceptions might themselves be responsible for engendering public distrust and, perhaps, impeding the recruitment of subjects for trials. Watch for someone to invent and then trumpet the following scenario: News reports of trial problems engender distrust; distrust impairs recruitment; recruitment woes are reduced by on-line trial listings; on-line trial listings overstate the benefits of participating in trials; reports of recruiting excesses engender distrust . . .

Clinical trial investigators, like all scientists, are often infuriated by others' doubts and criticism. But it should be clear that many critiques are offered in good faith – and many of those offering the critiques are mindful of the benefits of a solid human research infrastructure. Prophylaxing against problems becomes a moral imperative because anything that engenders distrust will impede the research that has shown itself to be otherwise worthy of the receipt of tax funds and which has, for a half-century, helped to reduce suffering, lengthen life, and otherwise improve the human condition. Do not cut corners here. Failure or sloppiness at this level, at this early stage in the growth of evidence-based practice, risks catastrophic and self-destructive results.

Many of these concerns reflect empirical questions, and it will be as well if we include them and others on the agenda of programs to study ethical issues in human subjects research. Meantime let us make a number of general suggestions for posting clinical trial information on the Web:

(1) Present information about individual studies as "flatly" as possible – i.e., stick to the facts and present them neutrally. Even then, it might be appropriate to seek IRB/REC review of on-line listings (if, for instance, future research demonstrated that IRBs were up to this task and that it would be feasible to undertake this).

(2) Emphasize that clinical trials are experiments and not treatments. If we knew that they were safe and effective treatments, we would not have to enroll in a clinical trial to receive them.

(3) Make clear that experiments have risks, some of which are not known until after people are harmed.

(4) Do not imply that patients on trials do better than those not on trials. While this is sometimes true,[4] it is often thought to be the case that subjects are attended to more closely than other patients, and this heightened scrutiny is beneficial. But to cite this as a benefit is also to admit that institutions provide different standards of care and so are guilty of a favoritism that can become an undue influence for some patients when considering whether to participate in a trial. If heightened scrutiny produces better outcomes, then provide it for all patients.

(5) Make sure that patients, qua prospective subjects, include their primary health care providers in this decision making. As ClinicalTrials.gov wisely counsels, "Whatever method you choose, it is suggested that you bring your search results to your physician to discuss whether a clinical trial will be appropriate in your situation."

The creation of on-line clinical trial listings is a potentially valuable response to patient requests. With certain safeguards, the World Wide Web should mature as a valuable source of information about these experiments and so be beneficial to patients, health providers, and investigators.

Internet use itself as a target of research

We began by observing that the concept of valid consent was one of civilization's great accomplishments. This is true, but like many other verities, it will benefit from some hedging. For instance, do we really want to insist that the valid consent of individuals is a non-negotiable requirement for all research involving humans? If so, we have just rendered much epidemiologic research impossible and/or unethical, and psychology, sociology, and anthropology are on the rocks. What we actually do in such cases – at least with epidemiology and certain other kinds of research (perhaps including emergency medicine) – is defer to the notion of implied consent. This is the view that, all things being equal, most rational people would not object to the acquisition of data about them if certain conditions are met.

Failing that, we rightly insist on consent being obtained from an appropriate surrogate decision maker, for instance a parent in the case of a child or a spouse or good friend if the subject is mentally incapacitated.

Now, though, we encounter the phenomenon of the Internet and Web themselves becoming sites for scientific observation and intervention. It is a belief of the greatest importance in evidence-based medicine that these sites should be patient centered and address patient values (Sackett et al. 2000). How shall we do this, given the importance people attach to health questions that are unlikely to be answered by a randomized controlled trial?

To illustrate, try the following: Type "PTSD" (post-traumatic stress disorder) and "chat" into your favorite search engine (or, perhaps, "(your city)," "AIDS," and "chat"). The result will be the usual mishmash that results from browser searches, with the following interspersed throughout: chat rooms in which Vietnam Veterans and others (in some cases their spouses and/or significant others) discuss personal experiences with PTSD. In some cases one needs to register to join the chats, but in others the chats and their archives are out there for all to see. What sort of privacy protections apply to this kind of personal behavior in cyberspace? How does it differ from similar behavior in traditional forums?

Now consider the issue of public health surveillance and intervention. A syphilis outbreak occurs among gay men who met sexual partners in an Internet chat room; public health officials used case-control study methods to determine that meeting partners on the Internet was "strongly associated with acquisition of syphilis" (Klausner et al. 2000). This information was then used to perform partner notification. More generally, people who use the Internet to find sex partners are, according to at least one study, "more likely to have concomitant risk factors for STD/HIV than clients who did not seek sex on the Internet. Thus, seeking sex on the Internet may be a potential risk factor for STD/HIV" (McFarlane et al. 2000). Does this place a duty on public health officials to monitor on-line meeting places?

Most generally, what rules should be followed by scientists hoping to observe, record, and otherwise study such behavior? How precisely does valid consent apply in cyberspace?

Heisenberg effects

In both examples here – chat rooms for discussing issues in personal mental or behavioral health and for finding sex partners – the very act of obtaining consent would alter the environment one is studying: Participants in the chat rooms are more likely to cloak, move, or otherwise alter their behavior if they know (or suspect?) they are being observed. We might call this an "Heisenberg effect" after the famous and related phenomenon in quantum physics, wherein the act of observing a system alters the system, thus corrupting or at least altering it as a research venue.

Scientists drawn to chat rooms as research venues are therefore in a pickle, at least if valid consent is a requirement for gathering data. Either they violate that requirement, or they ruin their observations.

The question for us is whether the concept of implied consent might, as above, provide adequate license for proceeding with the research in environments in which explicit consent would be a state-of-nature corrupter.

Psychologists and others have long grappled with the problem of deceiving subjects about the existence or point of certain research. The ethical permissibility of any such deception will be a function of: the level of risk to subjects, the value of the research to the subjects or their communities, the degree of IRB oversight, the extent to which the research requires violations of privacy, and whether the community being studied can expect any benefit from the research.[5] In the new world of on-line research, we are only just beginning to get a handle on the kinds of rules that might apply. In the absence of a clear and present public health emergency, though, there are a number of ways to proceed.

Consent vs. disclosure

The health of citizens in open societies is regularly observed, measured, and evaluated. The citizens permit this, we may presume, because they recognize the benefits that follow from such monitoring. It is just as well: Individuals are not given the right or opportunity to opt out of certain kinds of data collection. (Imagine parents insisting that their new baby's birth should not be recorded among the society's vital statistics, or that grandmother's death should not be recorded.)

The question of on-line behavior research will vex us until we have a better sense of precisely what benefits will follow from it and of how much privacy we have to give up to enjoy those benefits. Certainly, the benefits must be evaluated across all of society and not just among those in the chat rooms. It means we must weigh individual rights against collective goods – and our scales have yet to be tested in cyberspace. Still, there are important indicators that at least some research can proceed in an ethically optimized manner.

For instance, the Web is already widely seen as blurring or even collaps-ing the distinction between public and private discourse, and many people (perhaps mostly researchers!) regard the Web as a fundamentally public medium (Siang 2000). No matter where one sits and types, the digitized messages are often transmitted and available around the world. Further, public health scientists studying the syphilis outbreak found that "A major-ity of the surveyed Internet users reported that outreach was an appropri-ate and helpful activity" (even as news reports of the outbreak prompted antigay hate messages to the chat room) (Klausner et al. 2000). And none of the occupants of the chat room was ever publicly identified.

This suggests at least the outline of a policy for on-line research:

(1) Disclose as a general matter that on-line research is occurring or a pos-sibility. This might parallel regulations for consent-free emergency research, in which institutions conducting such research must disclose to the community that patients in their emergency departments might be included in trials;

(2) Those collecting the data must be representatives of trusted organizations;

(3) The data will be used for a widely regarded good, such as improved public health;

(4) The data will be kept anonymous, i.e., at least publicly (and maybe in all respects) decoupled from individuals' unique identifiers (name, address, Social Security number, etc.); *and*

(5) Some oversight body (an IRB/REC) will be scrutinizing the protocol.

Of course, the idea that such requirements will simultaneously protect subjects and benefit the common good will require more experience to determine. Given the possibility of public good, however, it would be blameworthy not to try.

Databases

The future of biomedical research is computational. Indeed, we have already passed the point at which we could do, or keep track of, our science without computers. As above, this imposes apparently contrary duties: We have the duty to use computers, if doing so will help us conform to an evolving stan-dard. And we have the duty not to use computers in inappropriate ways. We can survey these duties by addressing personal information storage and various forms of outcomes research.

That evidence-based practice has been successful in entering and reshaping the current healthcare Zeitgeist may be attributed to work begun by John E. Wennberg and colleagues at Dartmouth Medical School more than a quarter-century ago. Research for the *Dartmouth Atlas of Health Care* makes use of stored health records and has shown that care in the United States varies dramatically by region, that effective care is under-used and ineffective care is over-used, and that expensive care is often emphasized and on the increase in spite of the fact that there is little or no reason to believe it will work (the literature here is large; see Wennberg and Gittelsohn 1973, 1982; Wennberg 1984; Birkmeyer et al. 1998; Center for the Evaluative Clinical Sciences 1999; cf. Redelmeier and Tversky 1990; Clancy and Eisenberg 1998). Among the more noteworthy findings are that the number of procedures for specific conditions in a community is based less on clinical indications than on the number of surgeons trained to do the procedures, and, independently, that surgeons who perform a procedure more often than others have better outcomes than others. The former is a key motivator for health reform and the latter is essential for informed or valid consent.

What this means for our purposes is that the evidence of outcomes research is essential for high-quality practice, and the patterns it reveals, while scientifically and statistically off a quarter of a turn from the kind of work that goes into systematic reviews, are necessary to demonstrate to clinicians that their "standard procedures" might either not work or be harmful, that (some of) their beliefs about practice efficacy might be false, and that they are duty-bound to attend to these data as part of continuing education. We can put this as strongly as we like: It is unethical not to make evidence from this level, as well as from the level of systematic reviews, part of daily practice.

Personal information acquisition, storage, and use

Let us catalog some forms of computational data storage, distinguishing among them based on their relation to future, current, and past research. These data are stored on office computers, organization or system mainframes or networks, or very large networks, including the Internet and World Wide Web.

- Pre-research data. This is information from clinical encounters, including patient "chart" information, pharmacy data, insurance and billing details, etc. We call it "pre-research" even though it might never be used for research.

- Research data. This is information collected or accessed during experimental protocols, observational and outcomes studies, etc.
- Post-research data. This is research data obtained after the completion of a research project, for instance after the publication of research results.

These categories are not rigid: Pre-research data can become research data when, for instance, an investigator includes the results of a clinical encounter in a chart review study, and research data, as noted, can become post-research data. And data might be in two or even three categories simultaneously, though we might not be aware of this at the time.

These categories and relationships are at least facilitated and perhaps enabled by computers. The use of personal information for research and clinical purposes is, of course, not new. What is new is the extraordinary facility and breadth of the kinds of uses to which personal information can now be put. Another way of making this point is by saying that information technology makes possible research that was perhaps not possible – and certainly not practical – before.

Each of the three categories raises different (sets of) requirements for valid consent, depending on who will use the information and what the information is about. We will call these "consent profiles." For instance, pre-research data are acquired during clinical encounters, for which we may presume valid consent was obtained, and in certain circumstances (see below) may, according to the consent profile, be converted to research data without consent, if doing so is approved by an IRB. At ground, the relation between consent and information is shaped by considerations of privacy and confidentiality. We presume that all personal health information should be kept confidential – not acquired, stored, or used – unless (1) the person whom the information is about consents to its disclosure (as to an insurance company, a researcher, or another health professional), or (2) there is an ethically adequate justification for sharing, releasing, or disclosing the information in the absence of such consent.

We use the term "information" with some glibness, despite the fact that it is actually quite broad and might not accomplish the tasks we are setting out for it. This is especially true in the case of "outcomes research." Consider the following three sets of data:

(1) Jane has a head cold. She probably contracted it from her 4-year-old daughter, who attends a day-care center.

(2) Jane has HIV. She probably contracted it by sharing needles with other injecting drug users.
(3) Jane has cancer. She has it in part because of a genetic predisposition she shares with a number of family members.

Jane might plausibly feel free about sharing (1) with others, but not (2) or (3). And by "others" Jane might mean friends and (some) family members, but not government, corporate, or university researchers.

These points will be made clear in an illustration. Figure 4.1 contains a Venn diagram, where "data type," "data user/recipient," and "data" are classes. Let us stipulate that the intersection of the three classes contains the consent profile. This will help us to sort out the various issues that will arise as we move among different forms of information-processing research.

Outcomes research

There is not a clinic, practice, hospital, nursing home, hospice, or any other sort of facility where health care is provided that does not need to see how good a job it is doing. We can put this as broadly as we like: Outcomes research is the effort to measure the consequences of actions in health care. Or we can put it narrowly: Outcomes research is the effort to find out whether a particular intervention worked in a particular place (or, between the extremes, if it *tends* to work).[6] From hospital accreditation to managed care evaluation to quality assessment and improvement to the demands of evidence-based practice, outcomes research helps to inform us whether our labors make any difference, whether it is a difference we desire, and whether any of it is worth the cost. It is an information-intensive enterprise and it poses special challenges for the consent process. It is locally driven evidence-based practice, and it is often conducted by people who have no idea what they are doing.

It began, of course, with the work of British statistician and nurse Florence Nightingale (1820–1910) and her systematic data collection and analysis, which showed that improved sanitation would save the lives of hospitalized soldiers during the Crimean War. Her reforms, including the advocacy of data collection and analysis, met opposition – can you imagine it? – and it took epistemological cudgels on the order of "Those who fell before Sebastopol by disease were above seven times the number who fell by the enemy" to prevail (University of Minnesota 2001). The idea that these data could be collected

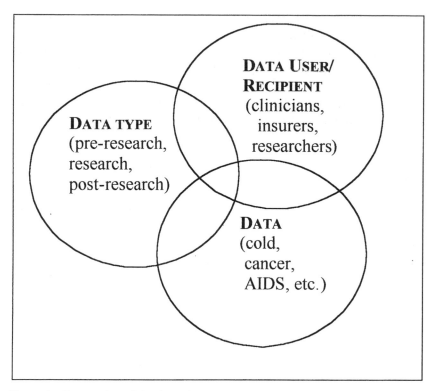

Figure 4.1 Intersection of the three classes

and that doing so mattered was embraced and advanced by Ernest Amory Codman (1869–1940) and his self-published *Study in Hospital Efficiency* (Campazzi and Lee 1997), and by the modern dean of outcomes research, Avedis Donabedian (1919–2000), whose book on outcomes and quality set the stage for much subsequent work (Donabedian 1980).

Quality assessment and improvement

Hospitals and related entities are under extraordinary pressure to demonstrate the efficacy of interventions, procedures, care plans, and so on and on and on. Without such evidence, it is reasonably argued, there is inadequate warrant to reimburse, reward, or otherwise salute the interventions, procedures, etc. This has led in a comparatively short time to a vast number of health professionals examining a burgeoning amount of patient data. As before, they are not tracking these data on 3-by-5 cards, but on computers. Rarely, if ever, however, do patients have any idea that people not directly involved in their care are regularly examining their personal health information.

Is consent required for this kind of use of patient information? In terms of the concepts and categories we have identified so far, this question may be put as follows:

> Is consent required for anyone to access Jane's file to transform pre-research data into research data for the sake of improving patient care?

Let's begin with the observations that: (1) it is not only Jane's file they seek but all files, or all of a certain subgroup; (2) it would be logistically impossible to obtain consent from all patients for all such investigations; (3) the survey is for the purpose of improving patient care in general; and (4) neither Jane nor any other patient will be identifiable in the conduct or the results of the survey.

Now we can ask whether these points constitute, as above, an "ethically adequate justification" for forgoing consent. It seems there are good utilitarian grounds to believe that they do provide such a justification. In striking a balance between confidentiality and consent, it would be unfair to many of those who would benefit from the research to insist that point (2) above be disregarded in the interests of a strict stance on confidentiality. This is especially so given the gist of point (4). If nobody can be identified during, or as a result of, the inquiry, it is not clear whether we are talking so much about confidentiality as about the desire or right to control information about oneself.

Here, it should be emphasized, is one of those places where information technology might provide solutions to the very problems it creates. If our ability to do a generalized computer query of a patient database puts us in a quandary about consent, then the structure of the database and query format should *themselves* be able to help reduce the ethical tension. They can do this by eliminating any unique information from the reports that will be generated in response to the query. Look at it this way: In pre-computer days, a hospital staffer who wanted to evaluate the efficacy of a procedure would have to pull the charts of all patients who underwent the procedure. Whether the staffer wanted to violate confidentiality or not, she or he would have a particular patient's chart in hand (with the patient's name on the cover). With an appropriately constructed database of all patients, however, it is possible to perform a query without ever seeing a patient's name, Social Security number, or address.

In other words, a computer might help us anonymize patient information and thereby reduce the need for consent. To the extent that this is the case – and it is increasingly the case – then it becomes blameworthy *not* to be able to perform such an anonymous database query.

We should in this context pause to note that some computer scientists are studying ways of using what we call "surrogate data ensembles" to identify individuals based, not on names or other unique identifiers, but instead on concatenations of diagnosis, birth date, postal code, etc. What this means is that the concept of "anonymization" is somewhat more complex than we might initially have believed. Contrarily, the same work that uses surrogate data ensembles to pick out individuals has a flip side, namely the use of correlate algorithms to protect confidentiality or safeguard it from computerized identity reconstructions. This is an area in need of much more empirical research, but the possibility that computers might be used to subvert – and better protect – confidentiality must be acknowledged (Sweeney 1997; Malin and Sweeney 2000).

Valid consent and confidentiality were never intended to impede credible strategies for improving patient care, especially if risks are low or absent. To the extent that computers themselves can eliminate risk (of stigma, bias, discrimination, etc.) then, we will have made substantial progress in adopting the tools of information technology in the service of patient protection.

There is another option that can be made a part of many consent profiles, namely disclosure to prospective patients of intent to survey personal information. Disclosure provides in some cases for a kind of truncated consent – the kind that comes from being able to opt out of a situation in which there occurs an activity one finds objectionable. So if Jane were contemplating admission to Hospital XYZ, she would be told in advance of the hospital's policy of gathering data for quality improvement. If Jane did not want her personal information to be used in such a way, she could choose not to be admitted to that institution. Such a "take it or leave it" approach will seem less than accommodating, especially if it turns out that all or most institutions adopt similar policies.

It is surely the case that computers could be used to decouple identifiers from hospital records, say, enabling research on anonymized data such that consent might not need to be explicit and applicable to specific studies. That is, we will do well to imagine and study the possibility that computers, in conjunction with a comprehensive policy of disclosure, could be used in support of a research program that reduces the need for consent by increasing the level of anonymity.

The requirement to disclose the intention to use data or obtain consent is embodied in current privacy and confidentiality regulations under the UK Data Protection Act and the more recent US Health Insurance Portability and Accountability Act. Both are fair attempts to strike balances between confidentiality and consent on the one hand and the need to do outcomes research on the other. Here, as elsewhere, there will be many opportunities for refinement, policy development, education, and ethical optimization.

Health services research

It will be useful to distinguish between "internal" outcomes research, as within individual hospitals, and "external" outcomes research, as occurs either within a single institution or across several but where the intent is to contribute to a broad or scientific understanding of outcomes phenomena. The "Common Rule" that governs human subjects research in the United States distinguishes between research that produces "generalizable knowledge" and other kinds of research; indeed, the Common Rule does not apply to research that is not aimed at producing "generalizable knowledge." Specifically,

> Research means a systematic investigation, including research development, testing, and evaluation, designed to develop or contribute to generalizable knowledge. Activities that meet this definition constitute research for purposes of this policy, whether or not they are conducted or supported under a program that is considered as research for other purposes.[7]

This has led to considerable debate about what precisely constitutes generalizable knowledge and, indeed, why protections should be lesser for people being studied for other reasons.[8] Those other reasons appear to include what we have here called "internal" outcomes research, for instance quality assessment and improvement.

Health services research is a larger domain and, indeed, one that in many ways is helping the drive for evidence-based practice, all the while seeking to balance the imperatives of consent and privacy (Institute of Medicine

2000). Health services research, construed in this way, is conducted by individual investigators, institutions, governments, and others. To the extent that the goal of those conducting health services research is to share the results, it falls within the scope of "generalizable knowledge." This means that such research must conform to the Common Rule. But the Common Rule permits waivers of informed consent for government research on public benefit programs and in cases in which:

(1) the research involves no more than minimal risk to the subjects;
(2) the waiver or alteration will not adversely affect the rights and welfare of the subjects;
(3) the research could not practicably be carried out without the waiver or alteration; and
(4) whenever appropriate, the subjects will be provided with additional pertinent information after participation.[9]

Of course, the waivers must be approved by IRBs or research ethics committees, which must document that the conditions in (1)–(3) are met. Using the tools of information technology to carry out this kind of research seems generally not to alter requirements of valid consent.

Knowledge discovery, data mining, and machine learning

In addition to storing information, computers – not humans using computers, but *computers* – can make discoveries and learn from the data. The idea that computers might make scientific discoveries, including discoveries of laws of nature, has been traced to 1958 (Newell, Shaw, and Simon 1962; Langley et al. 1987). This work has been of extraordinary scientific importance and has helped shape the evolution of artificial intelligence. Recent scientific advances (Lavrač 1999) should elicit strong interest among biomedical researchers because the tools being developed bid fair to change the way we think about research in clinical medicine, genetics, and epidemiology and public health. Knowledge discovery in databases, or data mining or machine learning, as it has come to be known, is, fundamentally, the use of computers to find useful information in large (sometimes very large) databases (Mitchell 1999; Mjolsness and DeCoste 2001). Some scientists are very excited indeed:

Where will this trend lead? We believe it will lead to appropriate, partial automation of every element of scientific method, from hypothesis generation to model construction to decisive experimentation. Thus [machine learning] has the potential to amplify every aspect of a working scientist's progress to understanding. It will also, for better or worse, endow intelligent computer systems with some of the general analytic power of scientific thinking. (Mjolsness and DeCoste 2001: 2051)

So, this is quite grand. More immediately, we are seeing new computer algorithms traversing vast amounts of information stored in connected databases and eliciting patterns and trends that bear on various research and clinical issues. Here are some examples:

- Bioinformatics. Knowledge discovery will be helpful to biologists trying to set up, maintain, and link or integrate sequence databases, and to help analyze expression data to identify biological function (Galal, Cook, and Holder 1997; Schulze-Kremer 1999). One can predict with confidence that some of the most exciting scientific work of the twenty-first century will take place at the intersection of computing and genetics, and in pharmacogenomics.
- Epidemiology and public health. From hospital infection control to data heterogeneity in environmental health, data mining techniques will provide powerful tools for making sense of large data sets (Brossette et al. 1998; Lamers, Kok, and Lebret 1998).
- Clinical medicine. In principle, all of clinical practice could be affected by database research. Data mining aside, health services research, clinical audits, and practice evaluation have led to calls – demands, actually – for more and better clinical data acquisition and storage (Black 1999). It might even be the case that database research methods will be able to supplement or augment data analysis from clinical trials (Padkin, Rowan, and Black 2001). Look also for knowledge discovery to inform the sciences of diagnosis (Doddi et al. 2001), prognosis (Richards et al. 2001), and hypothesis testing (Smalheiser and Swanson 1998).

Causation (again), uncertainty, and error

What is especially interesting in all of this is that no matter how brightly the sun shines on happy new sciences, there are nevertheless reasons to pause, to take stock, to question, to challenge. We began this chapter with a strong avowal of the power, utility, and success of applied ethics in the health sciences and professions. We can see here a new use for the discipline, as a sort of Eeyore to temper Pollyanna, although we needn't be gloomy about it but, rather, cautionary. This is because the data mining glass should, at least for a while, be regarded as half empty.

Consider first that many of the concerns raised in Chapter 3 about the absence of clear or direct causal links in meta-analysis and other meta-evidence apply also to knowledge discovery in databases. Analyses of machine-tractable databases[10] are re- (or, in a sense, meta-) analyses of data, and not direct or more immediate analyses of events or objects in the world. This is not to say that we ought to dismiss this work or its potential future clinical applications; that would be facile and stupid. It is rather that we should be insisting that, in our many and varied quests for biomedical evidence, we are simultaneously looking over our own shoulders. Relatedly: We have a difficult enough time identifying errors in ordinary evidence, and statisticians have long warned us that poor quality data ("garbage in") will lead to poor and inaccurate analyses ("garbage out") (e.g., Mosteller and Tukey 1977), and that data mining in particular offers exciting new opportunities for statistical misadventure (Good 2001; cf. a classic argument against allowing databases to replace clinical trials, i.e., Byar 1980).

If there is a theme, or a thread, here it is that of uncertainty. The reason we give pause at the threshold of knowledge discovery is the same as the one we give in seeking out differential diagnoses or in insisting on vast engines for education and research. It is a reason based on what has been called "the central role of uncertainty in all of medicine" (Szolovits 1995), and it is a call not merely for caution but for action to reduce or at least manage the uncertainty. If we are to reduce uncertainty, then making medicine evidence based requires that we go to great lengths to ensure that the evidence we are touting is worth it, and that the evidence we are rejecting was not worth, well, dying for.

Emergency public health informatics

There is an exquisite tension in the human subjects research and public health communities between data acquisition for research (recall the discussion earlier regarding "generalizable knowledge") and data acquisition for practice, be it quality assessment, public health surveillance, or whatever. The distinction is important conceptually because we reckon that human subjects are entitled to protections above those afforded to members of a community from whom we presume consent for public health and welfare data collection. In the latter case, society or the government is providing a *service*; in an open society, the credibility of the service provider warrants the presumed consent of those receiving the service. It is also important for those US institutions coming to terms with data protection under the Health Insurance Portability and Accountability Act. If I have HIV, say, and this information is reported to my local health department (which then commences the task of partner tracing and notification), then we see a case of public health in action. If, however, that same information is anonymized and placed, in aggregate, in a report that is then published, I have somehow become a subject in a research project.

This tension has never been greater than in the case of efforts to design, build, and test early warning systems for a bioterror attack. These efforts – dramatically accelerated by the suicide skyjackings and anthrax attacks of 2001 – provide an urgent testbed for data mining technology and the kind of evidence it provides. Let us call this new science "emergency public health informatics" and consider a case study to help draw out the more interesting and important issues.

A case study in early warning for bioterror

A government in a democracy is worried about bioterror attack. It seeks to support development of early warning technologies to reduce harm from such an attack, specifically to "develop, test, and demonstrate the technologies necessary to provide an early alert to appropriate . . . emergency response elements of a release of biological agents, involving both natural and unnatural pathogens, against military or civilian personnel." The project will require using data from government and commercial health databases ("while maintaining patient privacy privileges"). These could include hospital emergency department records, 911 telephone calls, certain pharmacy and supermarket purchases, etc.[11] (DARPA 2001)

This effort is, alas, a rich source of ethical issues. It is as well, then, that the epidemiology and public health communities have generally done a good job in putting ethical issues on their agendas, and there is a growing literature to provide orientation.[12] One ethical issue is obviously that of protecting privacy and confidentiality – or, more accurately, balancing privacy and confidentiality protections against benefits to be hoped for from the kind of ubiquitous data collection that such surveillance systems will require. (It might or might not be noteworthy that the government call for proposals refers to "privacy privileges." Given that the data to be collected could include those from emergency departments, supermarkets, and pharmacies, some might be inclined to regard protection of that information as a right, not a privilege. This is not to say that the information ought not be used in emergency public health informatics, only that the standard bar for doing so should be higher than for protections applying to privileges.)

Everyone agrees that, whether privacy is a right or a privilege, an individual who freely agrees to share personal information cannot be said to have been wronged by the sharing. The question that follows is whether such consent must be explicit or may be implied; whether, given the potential benefits, it will be adequate to obtain "community consent"; and whether it will be possible to develop adequate "trusted broker systems" that would allow personal information to be collected, anonymized by trusted intermediaries, and then shared with scientists (Wagner et al. 2001; cf. Merz et al. 1997).

For our purposes, the case presented here raises an issue that transcends privacy and consent. It is this. Any early warning system must, to be most useful in reducing death and injury, detect hazards as early as possible. As the information flows in from the various sensors, sentries, and detectors, it will paint a picture whose details become clearer by steps. There will likely be no "aha!" moment in the early stages, just suggestions, trends, and increased likelihoods. This might happen over hours or over days, or longer. This is all to say that the early warning system will at least initially produce probabilistic warnings – the software that will mine through all the rock in search of the vein of public health gold will be analyzing evidence and delivering it to human decision makers who will need to decide whether and when to intervene, to sound an alarm, to take action.

Given further that inaction, or perhaps more accurately indecision, is blameworthy, we can see that health authorities in the period after the aforementioned attacks found themselves needing to take a stand, to make a recommendation, to issue a guideline on the matter of anthrax and even smallpox vaccinations. The initial recommendations that resulted were a mixture of risk minimization, adverse event avoidance, and scientific uncertainty (e.g., Centers for Disease Control and Prevention 2001). The point here is not to judge the recommendations – a very difficult if not impossible task without the recommendations being invoked and in some way followed or rejected in an emergency – but to note the following steps:

• Identification of a problem (possibility of smallpox attack)
• Collection of salient data
• Noting uncertainty where appropriate.

But there is not at the end of the document an answer to the question,

"What shall I do *now*?" There is no guarantee that a vaccination given to prevent a harm might not itself cause a harm. There is only the science – probabilistic, uncertain, complex science – woven around the potential need to make a decision.

This, in conjunction with the use to be made of data from an early warning system, might constitute the highest stakes ever in probabilistic health decision making. For, like any public health warning system, the challenge is to strike a balance between the error of premature warning or action (which can engender panic and – or, perhaps worse – future distrust) and the error of tardy intervention (which can lead to preventable deaths and injuries). It is a challenge shaped by precisely the same uncertainty that we have seen vex and madden clinicians, and we will see it confront policy makers. And it is, again and overarchingly, an ethical challenge.

NOTES

1 Cited by Smith (1992).
2 Merely for instance: Goodman 1998a; Anderson and Goodman 2001.
3 Food and Drug Administration Modernization Act of 1997, Public Law 105–115, 105th Congress. Section 113, Information Program on Clinical Trials for Serious or Life-threatening Diseases. Food and Drug Administration website. Available at http://www.fda.gov/cder/guidance/105–115.htm.
4 And delightfully documented at the TROUT (*T*raditional vs. *R*andomised *OUT*comes) website, maintained by the Cochrane collaborators at McMaster University in Ontario: "How do the outcomes of patients treated within randomised control trials compare with those of similar patients treated outside these trials?" (TROUT Review Group 2001.) The answer is that people on trials appear to have better outcomes than those not on trials.
5 That is, privacy can serve as a powerful trump card in evaluating some research. Imagine hidden-camera observations of all sorts of behaviors. Even if scientists could demonstrate that the research was low risk and even if it could be shown that the research might in some way benefit the study community, we can say for numerous protocols that an IRB would err in approving them. How privacy is weighed in such contexts is a complicated matter requiring a careful evaluation of the potential benefits of the research.
6 See Weinberger and Hui (1997) for an outstanding and too-often overlooked set of reports on the role and use of databases in assessing quality, outcomes, and cost of care.
7 45CFR46.102(d).
8 A better way to understand "generalizable knowledge" is as a justification of risky research that has little or no prospect of benefiting individual subjects (see 45CFR46.406).

9 45CFR46.116(d).

10 The phrase "machine tractable" is adapted from work in natural language process-
ing (Wilks et al. 1990) and is distinguished from "machine readable." The former is
intended to suggest that a database – think of a dictionary – has been rendered more
useful and accessible, so that one could use it to find, say, synonyms and citations or
information about etymology; the latter is a computer disk containing dictionary
entries and nothing more.

11 This is of course an actual case study drawn from a request for proposals from the
US Government's Defense Advance Research Projects Administration (DARPA). It is
worth hearing in more detail:

> In addition to traditional threats to our national security, our adversaries now possess the ability
> to disable our nation's infrastructure and inflict casualties on U.S. citizens at home and abroad.
> One of the most insidious threats to DOD [Department of Defense] civilian and military per-
> sonnel . . . is a covert release of an infectious disease. If effectively executed, such an attack could
> go unnoticed and infect a large number of our forces with fatal disease. For the individuals that
> survive, the quality of life, burden on the medical system, and impact on the local government
> and economy is immeasurable. Surveillance for covert biological warfare and biological terror-
> ist activities is needed to counter the threat. If an event occurs, surveillance is needed to iden-
> tify the presence of the pathogen or the initial indicators of disease as soon as possible so that a
> rapid response can be implemented . . .
>
> Traditional disease surveillance requires that an astute physician recognize disease and order
> tests to confirm the clinical indicators. Once the disease has been confirmed, a health response
> can be initiated. For a covert terrorist event, the delays associated with this process would result
> in unmanageable casualties. New sensor and information technologies are needed to rapidly
> identify disease in the population. The objective of this program in bio-surveillance is to
> develop, test, and demonstrate the technologies necessary to provide an early alert to appropri-
> ate . . . emergency response elements of a release of biological agents, involving both natural
> and unnatural pathogens, against military or civilian personnel.
>
> The Bio-Surveillance System program intends to demonstrate that it is feasible to 1) develop
> an integrated system using diverse military, government (federal, state and local) and commer-
> cial databases from geographically dispersed locations, 2) glean applicable data from these data-
> bases while maintaining patient privacy privileges, 3) analyze the data to discern abnormal
> biological events from normal epidemiology patterns and 4) provide alerts to the appropriate
> DOD emergency response infrastructure. (DARPA 2001)

12 For overviews, see Coughlin and Beauchamp (1996); Coughlin, Soskolne, and
Goodman (1977); for early work on occupational and environmental health ethics,
see Goodman and Frumkin (1997); Goodman (1998c); and on the "codes-of-ethics"
craze, see Goodman (1996).

5

Evidence at the bedside

There is nothing remarkable in being right in the great majority of cases in the same district, provided the physician knows the signs and can draw the correct conclusions from them.
                                                                    Hippocrates (1983)

Evidence-based practice imposes extraordinary obligations on ordinary clinicians. Not only must the individual monitor salient scientific developments, he or she must plot performance against that of colleagues. The obligation to adjust one's practice in the face of "outcomes data" makes ethical sense only if we demand greater familiarity with the scientific literature, an ability to evaluate this literature critically, a clearer sense of the validity of outcomes studies, and an understanding of research methods ranging from randomized controlled trials to meta-analysis. This is a lot to ask of folk who, they will protest, just wanted to practice medicine. Contrarily, the ethical duty to conform to some kind of evidence-based standard (as long recognized by the need for continuing medical education) makes it difficult to know how much weight to assign to such a protest. At the end of the day there is a patient, a body of knowledge, and a need to decide how to proceed.

Cookbooks, algorithms, and guidelines

Physicians, nurses, and other clinicians would do well to eavesdrop on one of the larger, more interesting, and long-standing debates in the philosophy of science. While the debate has ancient origins, its contemporary flavor and importance are rich and immediate. On one side of the debate are philosophers who argue that scientific theories are either true or false, that these truths are discoverable and knowable, that science progresses over time by the discovery of more truths, etc.; these philosophers are called scientific "realists" (where the term has a special sense that is different from the use in ordinary language). Opposed to them are the anti-realists, who reject those views, in part by arguing that it is one thing to believe that a theory works or is able to explain phenomena and quite another to say that that makes it true in the grander sense required by realists. I appeal to this debate because two versions of the realist argument seem to bear strongly on the question of evidence-based practice, especially that part that is reflected in the debate over the use of practice guidelines, and which ultimately bears on the problem of how to incorporate aggregate evidence in the care of individual patients.

One version of the realist's argument is simply that he or she can best explain why science has been so successful. Surely, the argument goes, science – astrophysics, biology, electrical engineering – would not *work* if the stories we told were not true or approximately true, or, in the other direction, the truth of our theories explains the success of science. The philosopher Hilary Putnam's famous "miracle argument" for realism holds that realism "is the only philosophy that doesn't make the success of science a miracle."[1] This is the second version.

Now suppose we should regard, as I believe we should, medicine and the other health sciences as being successful because physicians and others generally and increasingly have true beliefs about human physiology, mechanisms of disease, and so on. It follows that the rational clinician wants to get her hands on as much information that bears on the truth of her beliefs as possible. That information, remember, is named "evidence."

Now suppose further that this evidence is best contained, represented, or summarized in a document that reviews experiments, case studies, and other information. Assuming further that the reviewer did a good job at this, then it seems not to make very much sense to disregard the review. Indeed, all things being equal, failing to act in accord with the best evidence is in many respects just what we mean when we say that someone is behaving irrationally. So if the world were this simple and straightforward, one would not only seek out and prize such summaries, one would, if they are summaries of the best or most effective medical treatments, have a clear and affirmative moral *duty* to act precisely as they direct. And if this is what we are talking about when we (derisively) refer to "cookbook medicine," then we would have a duty to follow the recipes, and our protests would be – *should be* – met with an equally dismissive: "Tough: It is true. Therefore it works. Therefore you should follow it." It can be fun to fool around with cake recipes, but if the cookbook is for treating a sick patient, why on earth would one want to fool around?[2]

However, I have spent a lot of time so far worrying that reviewers often do *not* do a good job, and have made repeatedly clear that medical decisions are shaped by uncertainty and not the kind of unimpeachable statements as appear in a cookbook. Maybe this is the reason that so many clinicians seem to revile even the hint that rationality demands a particular course, given a particular patient with a particular malady.

The "New Skepticism"

Recall from Chapter 2 that we, at one point, found ourselves in "something of an epistemic or communicative pickle" and laid out four ways or stances to take regarding the amount and reliability of clinical information:

(1) there is simply too much useful information to process successfully; or
(2) there is not too much information, but it is too difficult to find or separate from that which is not useful; or
(3) purported sources of reliable clinical information are in some way flawed or corrupt; or
(4) the amount of useful clinical information is tractable and reliable, and there are means for identifying it in the midst of non-useful information.

We may take (1), (2), and especially (3) to be exemplars of what we will call the "New Skepticism" – a sort of response to the new evidence. Old-fashioned skepticism holds that, for one reason or another, knowledge is impossible, unattainable, or undecidable. There are many flavors of skepticism in the history of thought and they begin with the epistemological goofiness of some ancients. Heraclitus, recall, said that everything is in constant flux and so one could not step into the same river twice; Cratylus followed by insisting that since everything was changing, even communication was impossible, so he refused to discuss anything with anyone, deigning only to wiggle his finger to signify that he heard something – but that a reply would be pointless since everything was changing. Skepticism matured somewhat, however, and, by some lights, has served a useful role as philosophical challenger and underminer of dogmatism (Popkin 1967). That said, it is no substitute for being right.

At any rate, the evidence-based movement has engendered an opposition movement. Opponents of evidence-based medicine do not, of course, object to the idea that medical decisions should be based on (the best available) evidence. Neither do they usually identify items (1) or (2) just above as the source of their skepticism; the skepticism is not philosophical or based on the skeptics' (or general human) inability. The new skeptics distrust the evidence itself, or its sources, or those who would urge its uptake and application. An important attempt to study clinicians' reticence, hesitation, and disdain for outcomes data and practice guidelines identified three categories:

(1)   [S]kepticism about the source, reliability, and objectivity of outcomes data, including the validity of inferences drawn from the data to construct practice guidelines;

(2)   [O]bjections or hesitations based not on the reliability of the data or guideline recommendations but on contrary patient preferences, clinical experience, and legal worries; and

(3)   [T]acit motivation, rarely stated but apparent in the sociological literature and/or admitted hesitatingly by physicians [i.e., that colleagues were actually motivated by profit, ego, ignorance, etc.].[3] (Boyle and Callahan 2000)

There is no doubt a great deal of value in acquiring a greater and clearer understanding of clinicians' attitudes toward practice guidelines, critical pathways, and the other levers and pulleys of evidence-based practice. Indeed, the study and analysis of these attitudes have themselves come to constitute a kind of subspecialty in health services and sociology research. (See, for instance, Cohen et al. 1985; Lomas et al. 1989; Haynes 1991; Patterson-Brown, Wyatt, and Fisk 1993; Tunis et al. 1994; Cabana et al. 1999. Moreover, keep an eye out for the literature that measures – and disputes – effectiveness of efforts to overcome this reluctance: Adams et al. 1999; Freemantle et al. 1999; Gifford et al. 1999; Stross 1999). But there is something troublesome about the flavor and tone of this skepticism. Notice that some clinicians who distrust guidelines regard them as challenging their intellectual capacity, ignoring their clinical experience, and generally impeaching their medical authority and autonomy. Distrust of guidelines seems to entail disregarding them altogether.

The reasoning of the physicians played upon two issues. One of them is that there is a difference between statistical outcomes in general for a class of patients and what might be effective with a particular patient. Outcomes assessments are probabilistic; they do not guarantee what might be efficacious in individual cases. A second issue turned on the belief that clinical experience can discern and take account of more evidence than encompassed within the scope of outcomes research. At the heart of the complaint against "cookbook medicine" is the belief that it runs roughshod over clinical experience and the uniqueness of individual cases. (Boyle and Callahan 2000: 12)

This suggests that the issue at its vexatious best is not entirely that clinicians regard the evidence as flawed or corrupt, but that they use those reasons in justifying a robust defense of their professional autonomy. Evidence-based practice is seen as *demoting* human clinicians. Indeed, it is at precisely this seam that the sloganeer traditionally comes to the rescue by suggesting – or, nowadays, insisting – that medicine is an art as well as a science. The implication is that science alone . . . *mere* science . . . is inadequate to its awesome task. Hippocrates invoked art to augment evidence he did not have; we now invoke it to impeach the evidence we do.

Art vs. science

Consider any number of the cases, instances, or beliefs for which we (now) enjoy (nearly) perfect evidence: Germs (and not humors) cause disease. Antibiotics (and not Zeus) kill many kinds of bacteria. Antibiotics will not work on viruses. And so on and on and on: We actually know a great deal of biology, physiology, pharmacology, and so forth. We have resolved issues long in dispute, we have increased our ability to apply knowledge to reduce human suffering, and we have progressively improved the education of successive generations of clinicians. We have, that is, progressed scientifically. Where then is the art in diagnosing an infection and in prescribing an antibiotic? In resecting a tumor? In treating a head injury, kidney stone, or left-toe boo-boo?

Make no mistake: The point is emphatically not that the practice of medicine, nursing, psychology, or pharmacology does not require intelligence, insight, and even creativity in using and applying science – it is that if the science is strong enough, it is not clear what is gained by invoking art. And when the science is not strong enough, then crediting art with decision-making success may provide emotional succor, but it does not provide any sort of guidance for clinicians. What can "art" mean here, other than playing hunches, winging it, shooting from the hip, and getting lucky on enough occasions to convince us there is something substantial to it? More congenially, perhaps, is the idea that when we invoke art in clinical practice we are using the term metaphorically. If this is right, what we really mean is that a clinician in a tight spot has made the most of imperfect information or inadequate evidence. It could very well be the case that "art" in clinical practice is really just the skills brought to bear in making decisions in the face of scientific uncertainty. But if the intent in using the term "art" in the first place – and in setting it in frank opposition to "science" – was to suggest something ineffable, mysterious, or beyond rational analysis, then it is not clear how, or even why, one would want to endorse it.

Let us look at this from a different angle. Suppose a clinician has used evidence of high quality and unimpeachable authority and reliability to render a diagnosis and create a treatment plan. It would then be irrational for her not to act in accordance with this evidence. Yet we have plenty of examples in which clinicians do precisely that, as for instance in the many cases in which patients with viral infections are given antibiotics to avoid disappointing or angering them. Could it plausibly be contended by those prescribers that art underlay their clinical judgment? Of course not; they were responding to social and perhaps other pressures (a not entirely convincing rebuttal of the charge of irrationality, especially given the adverse public health effects of such a stratagem). But it means that art, whatever it is in these contexts, is no good except metaphorically for making decisions based on slender evidence, and unnecessary for making decisions when the evidence is sound.

Maybe what is really intended by "art of medicine" is the *creative* process that takes place when a human makes cognitive connections between and among (more or less) dissimilar facts or signs or rules. Well, this is inoffensive: Medicine, nursing, and the other applied sciences provide wonderful opportunities for creative work.[4] But we must take care not to confuse "creativity" with "intuition" or "hunch" or any other cognitive event that cannot be taught or learned or failed at. Another way of putting this is that the task of making inferences from evidence – inferences about diagnosis, prognosis, or best treatment – are eminently *logical.* But there is much more to clinical practice than logic and, indeed, we tend to like it that way: For many maladies, at least, Dr. McCoy is much preferable to Mr. Spock. John Lantos has made a similar point:

Medical science and medical practice overlap but are not synonymous . . . In addition to public health interventions, many medical treatments are so safe and effective that they have been taken out of the hands of doctors and given directly to the public . . . To the extent that science allows discovery of safe and effective treatments, however, the need for doctors diminishes . . . There were doctors long before there was medical science. Whatever these doctors were doing, they created a profession. Science is a relatively recent overlap upon a very ancient model. When I, as a modern doctor, make a clinical decision for a particular patient in a particular situation, I need to integrate knowledge about biology, pharmacology, and pathophysiology with knowledge about psychology, communication, economics, and sociology, and with beliefs about morality, loyalty, and friendship. Scientific knowledge is a part of my decision-making process but often not the greatest part. (Lantos 1997: 154–5)

This seems right. An effective physician is not necessarily a logician; a good nurse knows about things from outside the realm of nursing science; a competent psychologist can navigate well by virtue of skills different from those directly related to behavioral health. But none of these observations counts as a reason to discount or set aside the duty to practice evidence-based medicine with individual patients. Either the evidence is valid, in which case you must attend to it; or it is not, in which case you have to act based on some sort of reason; or you just do not know, but need to decide on a course of action nonetheless. "Art" will not help you here – neither hunches, guesses, nor intuition.[5]

It has been suggested that we should think of the science of medicine as *quantitative*, and the art as *qualitative*, or based on text and not numbers and so as "applying procedures for interpretation of meaning instead of statistics to calculate probabilities, aiming for wholeness rather than details…" (Malterud 2001). This is perhaps a celebration of "clinical intelligence" and "clinical expertise," which are not so much defined as set in opposition to "outcomes-based behavioral regulation" (Tanenbaum 1993). But we can make qualitative research evidence-based as well, with findings from this research-enhancing "awareness of social dynamics in the clinical setting" (Giacomini and Cook 2000: 481). It seems that there is just an urge, perhaps a metaphysical longing, to keep some aspects of medicine off limits to reductionists, materialists, and others who insist that medical practice and the behaviors of clinicians can – because they occur in the world, in *this* world – be available for analysis. But no matter how often or how far this barrier is moved, no matter how thick the desired curtain between quotidian practice and the ineffable genius of the clinician, as soon as we peer behind it we see someone in a lab coat, doing science.

Practice guidelines

Here is a handy clinical guideline for the plague:

When there was a most cruel pestilence at Montpelier, in the year 1630, when they were infected with the Plague, they sent to me to know what they should do. I remembering that I had read . . . that the pickle of those little fish called Anchoves, had helped some of the Plague. I advised them to take thereof. One Patient drank a porrengerful by it self, another took it mingled with urine, and both were cured, for there followed vehement evacuation both by vomit and stool. (Culpeper, Cole, and Rowland 1678)

Apart from the splendid idea that anchovies might have medicinal properties, the point of citing this "famous and rare cure" is to underscore that the entire history of medicine has, in a number of interesting respects, been overwhelmingly about seeking and giving guidance. It is what happens in medical school, it is what goes on in medical text books, and it is what is shared at conferences, conventions, and continuing medical education lectures. Moreover, clinicians have traditionally *liked* guidelines, at least as long as they were not imposed by others, but sought out, like hidden prizes, in the mess of practice variation. Anyone who thinks otherwise should think about the popularity of clinical "pearls" and other suggestions, mini-algorithms, words of wisdom, sidewalk consults, and the like.

The point is made only to defuse some of the more vehement objections to the idea of clinical or practice guidelines. There might be a lot wrong with current guidelines, but the *very idea* of a guideline is something that is attacked or impeached at risk of extensive and serious self-injury.

Consider the National Guideline Clearinghouse – an extraordinary effort by the (US) Agency for Healthcare Research and Quality (2001b). The Web-based resource accepts the Institute of Medicine's definition of guidelines as "systematically developed statements to assist practitioner and patient decisions about appropriate health care for specific clinical circumstances" (Field and Lohr 1990: 39) and manages some 800 guidelines. Search for "otitis media," for instance, and you will find more than 20 more-or-less salient guidelines, from which you can select several for a side-by-side guideline comparison. It is like looking up something in a book, except that (1) it is up to date, (2) one can compare several books at once, and (3) it can be done quickly. Why would anyone disregard or ignore this resource? Actually, there are two distinct questions there. Consider first the Clearinghouse's disclaimer:

These guidelines are not fixed protocols that *must* be followed, but are intended for health care professionals and providers to consider. While they identify and describe generally recommended courses of intervention, they are not presented as a substitute for the advice of a physician or other knowledgeable health care professional or provider. Individual patients may require different treatments from those specified in a given guideline. Guidelines are not entirely inclusive or exclusive of all methods of reasonable care that can obtain/produce the same results. While guidelines can be written that take into account variations in clinical settings, resources, or common patient characteristics, they cannot address the unique needs of each patient nor the combination of resources available to a particular community or health care professional or provider. Deviations from clinical practice guidelines may be justified by individual circumstances. Thus, guidelines must be applied based on individual patient needs using professional judgment. (http://www.guidelines.gov/)

One might then choose to *disregard* the content of a guideline because it does not apply to one's patient. But one would *ignore* the resource completely because one believes that the guidelines will never, or rarely, apply to one's patient. The disclaimer recapitulates the history of the outcomes/evidence/guideline debate:

I believe that this treatment will help this patient.
Why?

Causal forces are regular and the future will be pretty much like the past.
'Tis not. It just seems like that.

'Tis so. If we do experiments and carefully observe events and their sequelae we can determine what tends to work.
"Tends to work" is vague; someone needs to make sense of it all.

Fine, our experts will provide reviews of the experiments.
But your experts are biased and subjective.

Fair point. We will apply the scientific method to these syntheses.
Your syntheses are based on sloppy, conflicted and contradictory experiments.

OK, we will do a better job of it, and organize these syntheses – better to identify shortcomings in the experiments.
Even so, now there are just so many different things to keep track of.

Then we will pull together statements that summarize the information and make it useful in your clinic.
Ah, so I should believe that this treatment will help this patient?

Actually, no, these guidelines are not fixed protocols that *must* be followed, but are intended for health care professionals and providers to consider . . . (http://www.guidelines.gov/)

The gist of this debate is of course replayed regularly in all areas of life, and has been a theme in logic and philosophy since the ancients. Under what circumstances should I embrace a belief? How can I be certain about it? What if I am wrong? What if my wrong action causes or allows my patient to come to grief?

Guidelines for guidelines

Had there been no attempt to "identify and describe generally recommended courses of intervention," we should say that something had gone wrong, even terribly wrong, with the very fabric of clinical science. Why – we should pose this as a question – why ever would one *not* want to have access to the experience of others, to the recommendations of others who have, as a matter of fact, spent a fair amount of time trying to craft and improve such recommendations? And why not do this well, collectively, and systematically (Campazzi and Lee 1997)? To be sure, rationality (not to mention the evidence-based canon) demands that the best evidence be used in patient care. But what has been called the "evidence gap" between clinical trials and individual patients (Mant 1999) afflicts us everywhere we turn. We must draw from the general and apply to the particular.

From the beginning of the current iteration of the guidelines movement (e.g., Eddy 1990b, 1991) it has been clear that we need to address and attempt to reduce this tension, in part perhaps by recognizing that medicine is a *practical* human science (Gatens-Robinson 1986). The idea of a guideline is that, at its best, it helps make practical the application of knowledge in a clinical setting. Guidelines of one sort or another, as our earlier excursus on the anchovy plague cure suggested, are part of the fabric of all decision making – part of the background radiation of a cognitive universe in which we need to think and, eventually, act. The ubiquitous and powerful mental action called "clinical judgment" is then nothing more and nothing less than the application of human judgment via guidelines to problems in the world (we should call these "guidelines with a lower-case 'g' "). It would be senseless to suggest that the application of judgment to the world could occur without some sort of support shaped by understanding of the causal chains we have been talking about for so long. It is not mystical, not mysterious, and not cheapened or corrupted by trying to make those connections better and more explicit. Of course with *clinical* Guidelines ("Guidelines with an upper-case 'G' ") the stakes are much greater.

That is, with clinical practice Guidelines it is especially nice if we get it right. This is not easy.

There are problems with some clinical Guidelines, their provenance, their creation, their structure. For one thing, some of them are just not very good (Grilli et al. 2000). For another, they may be mistakenly used to measure individual performance (Long 2001). Guidelines are themselves based on some uncertainty, which must be disclosed (Woolf 1998). They can be rendered so as to bully or pressure dissenters, who might, after all, have good reason to demur;[6] indeed, they may even be seen by some as punitive (Woolf 1993). They might conflict with each other, requiring further evaluation (precisely what we might have hoped Guidelines would reduce) (Granata and Hillman 1998). Guidelines sometimes perpetuate the "widespread illusion of the single answer" (Berg 1997). Some appeal to authority that is "ultimately lacking" (Ross 2000: 67). There is even a case, in France, in which formal complaints to a Fraud Squad have alleged improprieties by some guideline program participants (Hurwitz 1999, citing Maisonneuve et al. 1997).

But shortcomings and variations in Guideline development, structure, and authority are used not only to impeach the utility or validity of individual Guidelines, but to undermine the very idea that clinical practice might generally be made more scientific or rigorous. This itself is faulty science, a little like the creationist who urges a biblical account of the origins of species because real scientists disagree whether evolution occurred smoothly or in discrete periods of intense change. That the scientists might lack evidence to achieve closure is a poor reason to suggest that they should set aside the best available evidence, throw up their hands, and walk away. It is still a worse reason to doubt the truth of evolution or embrace the fatuousness of creationism.

So, if we are on the right track so far, the thing to do is correct course, not abandon ship. We are now seeing principles and guidelines for crafting and improving clinical Guidelines, including frank calls for across-the-board quality improvement (Shaneyfelt et al. 1999; Shekelle et al. 1999). It is possible to evaluate Guidelines with increasing rigor (Grimshaw and Russell 1993) and to locate them in the constellations among other aspects of evidence-based practice (Cook et al. 1997). Quite generally, the literature is noteworthy for the frank assessment of the accomplishments as well as the shortcomings of clinical Guidelines (e.g., Woolf et al. 1999), leading one authority to conclude that: "In the end, practice guidelines are likely to achieve their greatest good by expanding medical knowledge rather than as punitive instruments" (Woolf 1993: 2653).

Like our other tools, they can reduce, not eliminate, uncertainty.

Computers, guidelines, and decision support

So: Clinical judgment, often invoked as part of a bulwark to protect medicine from the regulators, financiers, and academic evidence fetishists, actually incorporates a form of guideline acceptance or rule following. That
being the case, it becomes irrational to insist that clinical judgment is
somehow in opposition to, or conflicts with, the best inclinations of those
who would craft and improve guidelines.

Why not, then, incorporate all these guidelines in decision support
systems or computer programs that analyze signs and symptoms, evaluate
laboratory values, and render a diagnosis, treatment plan, and prognosis?

In fact, practice guidelines are already lending themselves to computational applications, at least in some research contexts. This work involves:
using computers to help with guideline development (Sanders et al. 2000);
information representation to ease interchange and sharing (Ohno-
Machado et al. 1998); development of a guideline representation formalism,
authoring environment, and execution environment (de Clercq et al. 2001);
and guideline management, including integration into clinical practice
(Terenziani et al. 2001). But closer relationships are possible, and they
suggest opportunities to mechanize guideline use and implementation
(Dayton et al 2000; Durieux et al. 2000; Mikulich et al. 2001).

Why not, then, to recast the question, allow computers to make clinical
decisions? What if computers produced *better* outcomes than human clinicians?

Indeed, for many applications they already do, and it is arguably blameworthy not to use them. Can anyone seriously defend paper patient records
and postal services as the best ways to store and transmit patient data?
(Similar questions could be cast for computer systems used for clinical
reminders, consultation, or education.) This and related arguments have
been made on a number of occasions, almost always in the context of a discussion of the ethical issues surrounding decision support software (originally Miller, Schaffner, and Meisel 1985; more recently, Goodman and
Miller 2001). What has also emerged from those discussions, however, is a
clear and nearly unequivocal opposition to allowing computers to trump
human decision makers. This opposition stems neither from concern for
conceptual turf in a human-machine rivalry nor from esthetic opposition
to the idea of intelligent machines making important decisions. It is based
rather on the recognition that human intelligence is better suited to the task

of diagnosis, say, than machine intelligence. Nothing sentimental here: Decision-support machines and software just cannot take care of patients, cannot know and understand patients the way humans do, and cannot make clinical judgments (Miller 1990).[7] It would be a mistake to confuse human intelligence with machine intelligence here, no matter how well the latter did on the test:

What is wrong is that the practice of medicine or nursing is not exclusively and clearly scientific, statistical, or procedural, and hence is not, so far, computationally tractable. This is not to make a hoary appeal to the "art and science" of medicine; it is to say that the science is in many contexts inadequate or inapplicable: Many clinical decisions are not exclusively medical – they have social, personal, ethical, psychological, financial, familial, legal, and other components; even art might play a role. While we should be thrilled to behold the machine that will make these decisions correctly – at least pass a medical Turing test – a more sober course is to acknowledge that, for the present at least, human physicians and nurses make the best clinical decisions . . . . (Miller and Goodman 1998: 111–12)

Another way of putting this is that clinical judgment, appropriately girded, is of far more use to the anti-algorithm forces than it was when it was being inappropriately deployed against practice guidelines. Humans and human judgment will prevail here, but it will be in part *because* of evidence-based medicine and its accouterments, not in spite of them. Computers, guidelines, and all the evidence in the world are *tools* to be used by humans seeking or needing a little more leverage in their clinical tasks.

A comprehensive, point-of-care, guideline look-up service linked to the best available decision support system with access to a very large database is still not practicing medicine. It might be, however, that one day a human without these tools will not be practicing medicine either.

Evidence and managed care

In the United States, at least, evidence-based practice has shown up at the door with its poor relation, managed care, and this has caused some tension in the family. That they are traveling together makes sense: Evidence-based practice may be understood to be saying that more and better education, data, guidelines, and the like will improve quality and outcomes; managed care says pretty much the same, but with the explicit goal of reducing the cost of health care. Given the ridiculously high cost of health care in the

United States, this is a not-unreasonable goal. The problem was that managed care in the 1990s was desperately mismanaged, with physicians being (1) enrolled on managed care "panels" from which they could be removed without cause or reason, and which imperiled continuity of care, (2) humiliated by having to appeal to nonclinicians for permission or authorization for specific procedures, (3) subjected to gag rules under which they could not discuss (more expensive) treatments with patients, and so on. Managed care has since shifted from the "Mother, may I?" approach to obtaining authorization for individual procedures, to a population-based approach – whereby one's performance is evaluated in comparison to that of colleagues and over time; it is then that outliers are punished, perhaps by being removed from a panel, and team players are rewarded, in some cases with cash bonuses.

In principle, a system of incentives to reward more efficient health care delivery, reduce waste, and lower costs could look something very much like a system that celebrates evidence-based care. Why do – or why pay for – something that does not work? Indeed, it has been suggested that managed care is evolving simultaneously with a "new professionalism" that has as a key component "participation in an evidence-based culture" (Mechanic 2000: 107), and that "we cannot understand managed care unless we understand its power as at least substantially due to its reliance on a claim to be better science" (Belkin 1997: 509).

Anecdote suggests that evidence-based practice enjoys greater support in the United Kingdom and Canada than in the United States (answering this question would inform a very interesting research project). A possible explanation for this is that the United Kingdom and Canada (and other countries) have not experienced the decade of managed-care acculturation that colleagues in the States have. That evidence-based practice is the culmination of centuries of scientific trends pales beside its appearance nearly contemporaneously with managed care. It was a bit of bad luck that Americans are still paying for. It also produced the sense, or illusion, for some in the United States that evidence-based practice would cut into their income, although, if true, this is likely to elicit precious little sympathy from their comparatively undercompensated colleagues in Europe.

At any rate, the practical efforts to bolt evidence to care management are themselves fresh, controversial, and evolving, doubtless producing new sources of data for future analysis: In one case, five health plans that cover almost every resident of Minnesota jointly developed 50 protocols or guidelines that were said to be applicable to as many as 80 percent of maladies that customarily result in visits to physician. The standardization of treatment will be effected by informing both physicians and patients of the care protocols, but physicians will not be required to follow them (Bureau of National Affairs 2001; Freudenheim 2001a). In Florida, a group of large employers agreed to provide financial rewards to physicians who meet certain outcome, cost, and patient satisfaction levels: "The goal is to utilize the information to reward physicians who have the best outcomes – pay for performance," according to the president of the employer coalition (Freudenheim 2001b). These developments may also, however, be read as using evidence-based culture as a politico-economic tool that helps promote a shift in power from physicians to payers and that:

. . . facilitates the work of medical managers. To begin with, evidence-based medicine reduces the discretion and autonomy of physicians. While in the past the authority of doctors prevented questioning of their clinical choices, with evidence-based medicine, payers and managers can ask physicians to justify their decisions, thereby reducing the clinical discretion of doctors . . . Moreover, when relying on evidence-based medicine, clinical choices are not justified based on clinical insight, medical training, or personal experience. Instead, they are based on data from journal articles in medicine, epidemiology, and economics, which rely on such analytical techniques as random clinical control trials [sic], multiple regression analysis, and cost-effective analysis. These methods don't require a medical education and place nonphysicians trained in social science, science, or public policy on par with physicians. (Rodwin 2001: 440 1)

What is wrong about such a view, beside the main point and the conclusion, is that it casts medical journals as remote, occult, even academic (in a pejorative sense). In fact, evidence-based practice is not merely or exclusively about attending to outcomes studies (from journals or other sources) or conforming to practice guidelines. It is about this week's *JAMA* or *BMJ* or *New England Journal of Medicine* or *Lancet*, and whether to revise one's beliefs and behaviors in light of them. The problem pre-dates systematic reviews and outcomes and guidelines in that *any* article can, in principle, create a tension about whether to revise a belief or practice. At its awful worst, managed care smoothes over detail that might be essential for high-quality care. At its outstanding best, it insists that such detail be placed in a community- and evidence-based context.

This produces a conflict between individuals and their communities, with the core question of evidence-based practice – how does the weight of evidence apply here, now, today, to the patient before me? – raising interesting questions for the courts.

Evidence-based practice and the law

Evidence in medicine and evidence in the law are completely different creatures. This might or might not be a problem, depending on whether the courts are asked to rule in cases involving evidence-based medicine. In fact, every case that has addressed the question of a standard of care or, more recently, "medical necessity," has been about the evidentiary support for a practice or action. This involves numerous malpractice cases. For our purposes, though, a more appropriate question relates to the role of evidence-based practice *as such* in the courts, perhaps involving the use of practice guidelines in malpractice cases.

Even so, we need to point to, set aside, or somehow avoid the problem raised by different conceptions of evidence. One should be forgiven some pessimism. The US Supreme Court, issuing what is arguably the most important scientific ruling in its history, *Daubert v. Merrell Dow Pharmaceuticals*,[8] made a philosophical hash out of different theories of evidence on the way to deciding that trial court judges are responsible for evaluating evidence presented in court (Foster and Huber 1999; Haack 2001). The head of the US agency responsible for www.guidelines.gov notes that, "The current debate over medical necessity and the definition of appropriate medical services highlights the conflict between the concept of evidence as it is used in the law and as it is used by healthcare experts. Epidemiologists warn that the absence of evidence of effectiveness is not tantamount to evidence of the absence of effectiveness . . ." (Eisenberg 2001: 372). Further, many of the most interesting, general, and difficult problems at the intersection of evidence-based practice and policy are normative questions, questions that require a value decision: "No amount of data can tell us the scientifically 'correct' priority to place on Viagra, or how much money should be spent to reduce someone's chances of fatal heart attack by 1 percent" (Morreim 2001a: 418–9).

Like evidence, method and theory in law are just different from method and theory in medicine. It is not clear what, in medical research, is most like, or analogous, to the law's conception and reliance on adversarial process. The law's incorporation of medical and scientific experts as part of the adversarial process does not thereby render medical and scientific expertise in general as similarly adversarial. Moreover, when it comes to practice guidelines, the very process of consensus building that shapes part of the process of guideline development speaks of a stance that is different from that required when assigning or apportioning blame.

Early speculation about the role that practice guidelines might have in malpractice litigation required that, for courts to have any involvement with them, they would need to be widely accepted in the medical profession itself (Garnick, Hendricks, and Brennan 1991). But determining "wide acceptance" is actually like identifying one of the prongs of a standard of care; what seems to be wanted, then, is a standard of care for determining a standard of care. We should perhaps look forward to one day enjoying the glorious spectacle of two experts disagreeing in court about the appropriateness of a clinical decision based on a meta-analysis and which had an adverse outcome (cf. Rosenbaum et al. 1999). Even among scientists, that could not be resolved without more information about clinical indications, alternative therapies, their comparative likelihoods of success and failure, etc. Indeed, the very fact that evidence reduces, but rarely eliminates, uncertainty is what keeps every bad outcome from being malpractice. (This point about fallibility will be very important for us in Chapter 7.)

Because practice guidelines are general and patients particular, it means that medical necessity, for instance, must be relativized to individual cases. But this means that the use of guidelines to establish culpability in actual cases will be difficult: While legal reasoning requires focusing on the facts of the case, guidelines are not about *this* case or *that* case at all but decision procedures to be followed – all things being equal (Matthews 1999).

In the United Kingdom, the "Bolam test" is "the standard of the ordinary skilled man exercising and professing to have that special skill,"[9] a stance that "enshrines a standard of customary care and clinical judgment informed by scientific evidence and professional experience" (Hurwitz 1999: 662). It follows that "Courts are unlikely to adopt standards of care advocated in clinical guidelines as legal 'gold standards' because the mere fact that a guideline exists does not of itself establish that compliance with it is reasonable in the circumstances, or that non-compliance is negligent" (ibid.: 663).

We are, notice, watching the medical and legal professions slumping in the same direction regarding the evidentiary status of practice guidelines in one respect: Both professions "are far from witnessing the day when guidelines can be conclusive and where following them diligently would preclude further inquiry into a physician's conduct" (Finder 2000: 116). Part of the reason for this is that there will likely never be a day when the guideline writers look up from their desks, conclude they have answered completely and truthfully all the questions that were before them, and knock off for beer. Neither the clinician nor the court in which he or she is being sued can wait for a kind of "final rule" or ultimate, dispositive account of what ought to be done – or ought to have been done in the case in question. "Participants in the court process," that is to say, "must present and interpret the law using today's knowledge. They do not seek exactitude or certainty because they cannot wait for definitive evidence to be developed" (Ferguson 1997: 21).

Professor Skip Rosoff has captured the tension between care at a particular bedside and general practice, with near perfect pitch:

The goal of effectiveness studies and [clinical practice guidelines] is not, despite what some physicians may believe, to remove all elements of discretion and professional judgment from medical care. There will always be the need – and, one would hope, the latitude – for the exercise of professional judgment. Still, as the body of what is knowable and what is known grows, the degree of latitude will inevitably be [affected] by the extant knowledge base. When one does not know what is right or wrong, everything is fair game to do. Knowledge brings limitations, or at least, the basis for limitations to be imposed. (Rosoff 1995: 375)

What follows from this is even more interesting. The law needs medical evidence to resolve cases involving medical practice. Medical practice needs better evidence. So as the evidence in evidence-based medicine improves, not only should medical care at the bedside improve, so should the courts' ability to resolve disputes there (Rosoff 2001)!

"Eraritjaritjaka"

A Belgian physician writing in The *Lancet* is mourning the way it used to be: More learning, more caring, more respect; no manikins or videotape; real clinical skills. So he confesses he has an increasingly bad case of "eraritjaritjaka." The term – it is worth sounding out – is attributed to novelist and philosopher Elias Canetti who, in his 1992 work *Die Fliegenpein,* reports it to be an "archaic, poetic expression in Aranta (an aboriginal tribe in Australia)" (Nauwelaers 2000: 2169).

To have *eraritjaritjaka* is to be "filled with desire for something that is lost." We hear this all over the place nowadays (the idea, not the word), although our predecessors probably always did, too. Still, there is something to the idea of a collective and cumulative loss of innocence as we move – as we progress – from the country doctor carrying his bag up a winding path to a farmhouse, to the clinician downloading clinical practice guidelines from a wireless network, to a personal digital assistant. Unfortunately there is no alternative to feeling *as* loss the change to more and hopefully better machines (although there is no need for us to have become rude in the process). But including "the way it used to be" among things from the past to be desired, as if the way it used to be were a lover or a hearth or a childhood home, is the path to madness. Progress is often austere, rarely accommodating, and generally indifferent. If it means, however, that healthy people stay that way, and that sick ones don't, then our longing becomes selfish and sentimental.

Evidence-based practice is neither a rear-guard insurrection by automata nor the latest clinical meddlings by pointy-headed boffins with nothing better to do than deprive clinicians of on-the-job satisfaction. It is an earnest and honest attempt to help clinicians do best what they already were committed to doing well.

NOTES

1 Putnam (1975); but see Leplin (1984) for a superb collection of papers on the realism–antirealism debate.
2 Note that in some information-intensive specialties, the availability of frank decision algorithms is welcomed, if not met with relief (cf., e.g., Morris 1998).
3 This noteworthy collaboration was sponsored by the US Agency for Health Care Policy and Research of the National Institutes, and carried out by the Hastings Center – the New-York-based research and education institution specializing in ethics.
4 Indeed, some opportunities are even "artistic" in an ordinary sense of the word. I am of course thinking about aspects of reconstructive, cosmetic, and dermatologic surgery and practice. Otherwise, there is many a brilliant, effective, compassionate, and creative clinician who could not see the need for, perform, or maximize the esthetic effects of, say, an H-plasty or some other kind of transposition flap. (I am grateful to Dr. Judith E. Crowell for this example.)
5 This includes "scientific intuition" and the like (see below). Either a cognition occurs in a human brain or it does not. If it does, it should lend itself to scientific scrutiny and produce public evidence. To argue this way is not even necessarily to debate the

mind–body problem or to take a stand on whether mental events can be reduced to physical events (or just *are* physical events); it is only to say that scientists give up the game by appeal to events (an intuitive decision, for instance) that cannot be measured or studied. This is not to say that the existence of such powers or forces is impossible, only that, like religious faith, they will not be governed by methods that we tend – with good reason – to defer to in the health professions. You might even find it in some way helpful, useful, or even perhaps efficacious to pray with your patients; Godspeed. But until you can identify which of some 4000 potential deities is helping you achieve this outcome, the ordinary rules of rationality and evidence will caution against prescribing it, teaching it to medical or nursing students, billing for it, or otherwise publicly expressing your support for it in an environment such that if you are wrong, your patient will die.

There are some who believe it is possible to make useful sense out of medical "intuitions," and they might be right, although I hypothesize that most physicians, including those who want to preserve a role for decision making with that *je ne sais quoi* element of genius added in, would blanch at their allies here. Consider the following:

"Intuition Medicine™ is a system of expanded perception of the world through the development of the human sense of INTUITION. This system . . . includes an integrated study of seven energy anatomy systems and their connection to the physical anatomical systems. This model of Intuition Medicine™ and its hypotheses have been synthesized from . . . intuitive counseling of thousands of people . . . This material and theory are not intended to be used in place of your doctor's advice. Rather, Intuition Medicine™ is intended to be used to increase the effectiveness of conventional diagnosis and treatment of your body, mind and spirit. (http://www.intuitionmedicine.com)

or

I disappoint some people when I discuss intuition because I firmly believe that intuitive or symbolic sight is not a gift but a skill – a skill based in self-esteem. Developing this skill – and a healthy sense of self – becomes easier when you can think in the words, concepts, and principles of energy medicine. So . . . think of learning to use intuition as learning to interpret the language of energy. (http://www.innerself.com/Miscellaneous/energy_medicine.htm)

6 Here is one especially vehement complaint:

Guidelines generate systematic and paternalistic pressure for the many to conform to the views of the few. They replace the gradual and time honored process by which non-specialists learn from experience with an attempt to force the pace of disseminating 'good practice,' measured by narrow criteria. The unquestioning pursuit of clinical guidelines without regard to the added problems and pressures they may engender poses dangers for us all, representing as it does the exercise of power without responsibility. (Haycox et al. 1999: 393)

7 If, in the future, computers could do all these things as well as humans, then it is sur-
rendering little to concede that they should be allowed – perhaps *required* – to do
them. Some ceremonies are worth standing on, and some are not. But it might be
that it will be impossible, given what we mean by the practice of medicine or nursing,
for computers ever to replace humans. The question is an old and unresolved one in
artificial intelligence; it need not detain us.

8 509 U.S. 579, 113 S. Ct. 2786 (1993). A number of soon-to-be-cited references are to
articles included in a very important issue of the *Journal of Health Politics, Policy and
Law*, the issue being based on a spring 2000 workshop jointly sponsored by the U.S.
Agency for Healthcare Research and Quality and the Institute of Medicine at the
National Academy of Sciences.

9 Bolam v Friern Hospital Committee (1957) 2 All ER 118–28, cited by Hurwitz
(1999).

6

Public health policy, uncertainty, and genetics

A skeptical farmer was raking leaves outside his barn when he saw a young woman from the city approaching. She carried a clipboard. "What are you selling?" he asked, almost rudely.

"Nothing," she replied. "I'm not selling anything. I work for the Bureau of the Census."

"What's that?"

"Well, I'm a census taker – we're trying to find out how many people there are in the country."

"Well," the man said, "you're wasting your time with me. I've got no idea."

Research syntheses have influenced policy and practice in areas as diverse as exposure to environmental tobacco smoke, mammography, and otitis media. In all these cases, decision makers – from individual clinicians to policy evaluators – have had to proceed in an environment shaped by empirical uncertainty. How, generally, can one ethically optimize a public health decision when one is unsure of the lay of the land? This chapter will identify these and other key policy questions, and address the problems that attach to the use of research synthesis to guide or inform public policy and legislation. As above, a number of very interesting case studies are available to illustrate this. We conclude with a discussion about a science – genetics – that will further challenge our ability to make momentous decisions in scientifically fraught environments.

Ethics and epidemiology

Epidemiologists are used to some of the kinds of epistemological problems we have been savoring. The question as to whether a pattern signifies a cause is as old as science itself; but when the question arises in the context of human health there is an extra-strong case to be made that we try harder to get it right. On balance and over time, it seems that humans have done an outstanding job in identifying causal relations and using that understanding to improve health and reduce suffering.

This does not mean that all individual decisions that contributed to that upshot were correct, only that, in aggregate, we've done a pretty good job of it. Now, this is actually too bad, because it means that any *individual* decision might have been wrong – and we wanted so badly to be right! Public health, policy, and epidemiology thus mirror clinical practice and, indeed, any other area of human inquiry: Any particular decision might be or might have been wrong. The task of inferring from the big picture to the instant case is often one of the largest and most difficult challenges we face. As I have argued repeatedly, though, it is a (large though simple) mistake to infer from difficulty to intractability, and as Chapter 5 showed, clinicians and others entertaining skepticism about the new evidence would do well to learn from the philosophical debate that produced the argument that the success of science entails the truth, or approximate truth, of causal theories. (Epidemiologists who are skeptics about causation would do well to review this debate.)

Recall from Chapter 4 our discussion of the use of databases in emergency public health informatics. Among the points of that account was that, even with a successful track record in using intelligent machines to help make inferences from stored information, it might be that, in any particular case, we will make the wrong inference. Coupled with the need to communicate to large audiences of wildly varying scientific sophistication, the difficulties multiply with rapidity. And, as we saw in Chapter 5, there are circumstances involving normative decisions in which no amount of data will solve our problems for us (although there might be circumstances in which more data will help, and in which morality would require that we gather more data). The task before us is to suggest ethically optimized strategies for making public health decisions in the face of empirical or scientific uncertainty.

It is also worth remarking that, while there is an evolving literature addressing general ethical issues in epidemiology and public health (see Chapter 4, note 12), there are vast opportunities to develop curricular tools and conduct research to advance work in the kinds of ethical issues we are considering here. A research and curriculum-development program that examined ethical and policy issues in meta-analysis and other systematic reviews would be a glory to behold.[1]

Evidence-based policy

At first impression, the phrase "evidence-based policy" should delight us with the same intensity as its variants have delighted so many in the research and clinical communities. It is so, well, *obvious*, that if one is going to make decisions and affirm certain practices and rules regarding and regulating the public's health, then one might as well have a look at evidence that bears on the questions on the table:

That politics is driven more by values than facts is not open to dispute. But at a time when ministers are arguing that medicine should be evidence based, is it not reasonable to suggest that this should also apply to health policy? If doctors are expected to base their decisions on the findings of research, surely politicians should do the same. Although individual patients may be at less risk from uninformed policymaking than from medicine that ignores available evidence, the dangers for the community as a whole are substantially higher. . . . As such the case for evidence based policymaking is difficult to refute. (Ham, Hunter, and Robinson 1995: 71, footnote omitted)

Perhaps we can come to regard – we *ought* to come to regard – the incorporation of evidence in policy as a form of "payback" by researchers to societies that have spent trillions in hopes of learning about the world and using that knowledge for human betterment. Research improves clinical care, and in the form of systematic reviews it constitutes payback on investments in research synthesis (Silagy, Stead, and Lancaster 2001). It makes no sense *not* to incorporate evidence in policy.

We might further suppose that collective policy and collective evidence are a better match than that which has shaped our course so far, that is, the match or fit between aggregate data and specific clinical circumstances. But this ignores the uses to which public policy is put – including guiding those same specific clinical decisions! It is as if the snake of policy has swallowed its tail of evidence, so that we no longer can tell where the particular and the general begin or end.

Moreover, the effect of research on policy is not clear, perhaps in part because either policy makers do not understand the research, or the researchers do not understand the needs of policy makers, or both. That suggests opportunities for future progress, however, by urging that policy makers become "more involved in the conception and conduct of research [and] Researchers need greater access to information on the priorities of policymakers . . ." (Black 2001: 278).

There is another concern, about research quality, and we must keep it front and center. We spent a fair amount of time in the first three chapters pointing out or documenting ways in which our science is not as good, honest, or reliable as we would hope it to be. We overcame any resulting inclinations to skepticism by calling for balance and appealing to the research engine's broadly positive and successful track record. Still, the application of research to policy should be seen to raise novel issues, especially regarding official or governmental responses to public misunderstanding of science. The voice of Alvan Feinstein was heard clearly in this arena, too, in the 1980s, when he noted the "epidemic of apprehension" produced by some cancer statistics reported as a result of "gross violations of epidemiologic principles and scientific standards for credible evidence" (Feinstein and Esdaile 1987: 113). The point, as fresh as ever, is that bad science will lead to bad policy. Alas, good science can lead to bad policy, too, but our hands are full just now.

It will be useful to identify a suite of case studies to illustrate the relation between evidence and policy. This will assist efforts to establish or at least sketch the kind of stance to be taken in making decisions in probabilistic environments that affect the health of communities.

Case studies in public health policy

Three cases follow, chosen for the sake of diversity in the issues they raise. Numerous cases are available to us, as perhaps is the number of lessons to be learned, but these three studies – on passive smoking, screening mammography, and otitis media – seem to cut nicely across the public health and policy spectra.

Case 1: Environmental tobacco smoke

It is clear, well known, and uncontroversial that cigarette smoking is bad for health; it is therefore a little surprising that secondhand cigarette smoke could provide so many opportunities for disagreement and controversy. It is surprising because, while it is possible that environmental tobacco smoke might not be harmful, it should occasion no great surprise when it is found that it is. Still, a nontrivial 37% of the reviews in one study (Barnes and Bero 1998) found that passive smoking is *not* harmful to health. (Lest we forget our own lesson, from Chapter 5 and regarding effectiveness of an intervention, we should be reminded of how it works in terms of epidemiological associations, namely that "No evidence of an association" is not the same as "Evidence of no association" (Stoto 2000: 352).) So, how could studies on the effects of passive cigarette smoking reach such divergent conclusions?

In January 1993, the US Environmental Protection Agency (EPA) classified environmental or secondhand tobacco smoke as a Group A carcinogen. This category includes radon, asbestos, and benzene, and is reserved for the most dangerous carcinogens (Environmental Protection Agency 1992). It was immediately controversial, in part because of its likely and widespread policy implications. *Widespread?* It is utterly breathtaking to observe the worldwide social and economic changes effected in the subsequent decade by restrictions on smoking in workplaces, restaurants, and airplanes. It is arguably one of the sharpest, quickest, and most thoroughgoing changes in health policy in the history of civilization.

The report is a key link in the chain that led to the following unequivocal statement: "Environmental tobacco smoke (ETS) is *known to be a human carcinogen* based on sufficient evidence of carcinogenicity from studies in humans that indicate a causal relationship between passive exposure to tobacco smoke and human lung cancer . . ." (Environmental Health Information Service 2001 (original emphasis)). Does it matter that the report was based in part on a meta-analysis of 11 US studies of smokers' spouses? That it excluded a number of studies done outside the United States (although it did include a number of studies from around the world)?

Well, this is low-hanging fruit, and it will be easy to wish for a large, randomized, double-blind, placebo-controlled trial while we pluck the existing results and carry them to the policy market. There is, that is, nothing to lose, at least in terms of public health. As it was put once, "Certainly it will break few compassionate hearts if the effect of a meta-analysis is to reduce the exposure of children, say, to tobacco smoke (Goodman 1998b: 160). Fair enough, but if one doubts the ability of research synthesis or systematic reviews to identify or tease out causal relations, then an over-hasty acceptance of such a tool might come at a price of reduced credibility. In other words, being right will not be adequate if word gets out that you didn't care about the methods. Feinstein again, passing on the remark of someone evaluating the consequences of the EPA study (1992): "Yes, it's rotten science, but it's in a worthy cause. It will help us to get rid of cigarettes and to become a smoke-free society."

To suggest that meta-analysis is "lousy science" might be to try to succeed by invective where reason and argument have failed, but the point is taken. We have a case in which scientific uncertainty – if it is that – has at its public health worst a policy consequence that will reduce the number of places filled with tobacco smoke. If only that were the worst consequence we find in applying the new evidence to issues elsewhere in public health.

Also, if there is a credibility gap here it lies with the investigators who failed to disclose their affiliations with the tobacco industry, or with editors and others who provided inadequate scrutiny in promulgating their work: "Our findings suggest that the discrepancy between consensus documents and published reviews related to the health hazards of passive smoking is primarily attributable to large numbers of reviews written by authors with tobacco industry affiliations" (Barnes and Bero 1998: 1569). Again, it is not science or method as such that are to blame, but ordinary human weakness.

Case 2: Screening mammography

If ever there were a debate over effectiveness that confused the public, angered clinicians, and caused evidence-generators to be held in less-than-high regard, it is in the sad and sorry case of breast cancer screening by mammography. It is an evidence-based catastrophe that ranges from the temples of systematic science, to government and insurance headquarters, to physicians' practices, to the living rooms of millions of women who, after decades of advice, must now worry that those who gave them that advice did not know what they were talking about.

It is not even clear where it began – the issue has long been shaped by controversy. We can start in 1997, when a National Institutes of Health consensus conference concluded that there was inadequate evidence to recommend for or against routine mammographies for women aged 40–49 years (National Institutes of Health Consensus Development Panel 1997). This led to an extraordinary official response, with Congress itself approving resolutions and calling special hearings on the consensus statement "to refute its conclusions and to give American women 'clearer guidance' about the need for mammograms" (Woolf and Lawrence 1997 (footnotes omitted)). In other words, at the nexus of science and public policy, it can sometimes make sense to be a champion or advocate in the *absence* of compelling evidence.

It gets better. Three years later, an ocean away, a key Cochrane Collaboration report concluded that "screening for breast cancer with mammography is unjustified" (Gøtzsche and Olsen 2000). The report, reviewing the quality of mammography trials and of a meta-analysis, as well as a new meta-analysis, said that "there is no reliable evidence that screening decreases breast-cancer mortality." This, too, led to "a storm of debate and criticism" (Horton 2001b), some of it surrounding the quality of the research.[2] This led to a formal Cochrane review that "paid close attention to the standard dimensions of methodological quality of trials . . . [and] found that the results confirmed and strengthened our original conclusion" (Olsen and Gøtzsche 2001: 1340).

But *this* has led to even more widespread confusion. Back in the United States, Barron H. Lerner, an internist and author of a book on breast cancer, is quoted in *The New York Times* as, in essence, throwing up his hands:

> The debate has become so sophisticated from a methodology viewpoint that as a doctor my head is spinning . . . you read an article in *The Lancet* and you nod your head yes. Then you read the studies by people on the other side and you nod your head yes. We're witnessing this fight between the pro- and anti-mammography forces and they're both arguing that "my data is better and we're right and they're wrong." (Kolata 2001)

What is dramatic here is actually something that happens quite often in science, but which is dissatisfying for those with little taste for uncertainty: Progress does not consist of the steady accumulation of truths but, rather, of a process of revision, purification, and re-evaluation. At the end of the day, or century, we know more than at the beginning, but this holds small comfort for many with low-uncertainty thresholds. Unfortunately, the confusion, disagreement, and controversy here are caused by the same systematic process we had hoped would give us clear warrant for all manner of clinical and policy decisions.

This was never supposed to happen.

Case 3: Otitis media

Otitis media (acute red ear, glue ear) is one of the most common diagnoses in children, with the number of doctor's office visits for the malady increasing more than two-fold between 1975 and 1990 (Agency for Healthcare Research and Quality, AHRQ, 2001c). The decision as to whether to treat the malady with antibiotics is simultaneously one of the most frequent and difficult ones pediatricians need to make. That there is a vast – a truly vast – amount of evidence has not made the decision any easier.

In the mid-1990s, a US Government study of thousands of articles and several reviews (Stool et al. 1994) was criticized for making recommendations of "dubious value" on the basis of expert opinion anyway (Culpepper and Froom 1995).

A query of the AHRQ's National Guideline Clearinghouse website using the keyword "otitis*" elicited 25 guidelines that address some or several aspects of otitis media and its clinical management. The first four were from the American Academy of Pediatrics; a Cincinnati, Ohio, children's hospital; the Institute for Clinical Systems Improvement (the Minnesota health plan consortium urging guideline adherence and mentioned in Chapter 5); and the US Centers for Disease Control and Prevention. Comparing the first and the last, using the website's side-by-side guideline comparison feature, produces the advice from one guideline that "Amoxicillin should be the first-line antibiotic for acute otitis media." The other guideline does not mention amoxicillin. More recently, an AHRQ-supported center study concluded that there is "no evidence to support the superior efficacy of any particular antibiotic or dosing regimen" (Takata et al. 2001).

Pediatricians are moderately familiar with the evidence for otitis media management, albeit with fewer than half noting familiarity with, or use of, applicable guidelines (Flores et al. 2000; they were somewhat more familiar with guidelines for asthma and hyperbilirubinemia).

There is a problem here and it is a kind of embarrassment of riches. We have a very common malady, a vast amount of research that has been synthesized by respected organizations, and an environment shaped nonetheless by uncertainty and, somehow, bitter disagreement among clinicians. In some respects, this issue is veiled from the patients and their parents, in part because the value of antibiotic therapy is so unclear. Indeed, it is possible that in some populations, children presenting with otitis media are prescribed antibiotics for no reason other than that the parents expect, request, and sometimes even demand such therapy. Either they do not care about the evidence or, if they do, they choose to manage their uncertainty by defaulting to the easiest and most familiar action – get a pill. That there might be adverse events associated with such a course (increased diarrhea, say) may be completely unknown to the parents; a physician could disclose the risk, of course, but only under pain of being met by an entreaty aimed at preventing him from doing nothing. Under such pressure, some clinicians will recall the lesson that they should have been taught early in their education, namely, "Don't just do something, stand there."

Lessons

The cases are instructive, although the lessons derived from such narratives may vary depending on which aspects have been highlighted. The decisions about what aspects to emphasize should be guided by some sort of shared or common interest, but there is room for variability here. Moreover, each of our three cases could be a book; each is a story about difficult decisions with high stakes by well-meaning people. The finer the granularity of the narrative, the richer and more complex the exchange. Indeed, books *have* been written about these issues, although apparently not focusing on aspects shaped by research synthesis or systematic science.

One thread that runs throughout the cases and which should be highlighted is that, when cases become policy controversies, there is a risk that some ordinary clinicians will close their ears to future synthesis or guidance. If I am right about the nature of scientific progress, then the problem with mammography screening, for instance, is a problem that may be viewed as part and parcel of the science behind many questions in disease prevention. We move, slowly and indirectly, from ignorance to knowledge, with uncertainty being our unhappy lot for much of the time. This is just the way it is. The proper and rational response to such a state of affairs is to soldier on, keep up with the literature, and learn more about how consensus is arrived at – not to throw up one's hands and conclude that the researchers are in perpetual error, and so may be ignored or disregarded.

That said, there is nothing like a conflict of interest or conflict of commitment to engender doubt. It is not only in studies or meta-analyses regarding passive smoking that corporate interests erode confidence in the results; pharmaceutical research itself has long been rife with actual and potential conflicts. Here again, the proper stance is to press on, as journals and sponsors largely have, to effect a course correction and get on with building or regaining reader trust. The experience with environmental tobacco smoke research sponsorship may be viewed in the following light: When research undergoes the process of uptake into policy, it provides an additional opportunity and means to cleanse the scientific corpus and filter out bias. It is a difficult and sometimes ugly process, but it may be preferable to the alternatives.

Among the lessons to be derived from the case involving otitis media is actually a reminder – that medicine, nursing, and indeed all of the health professions are practiced not in a vacuum, but in an environment shaped by interesting and complex social, economic, cultural, and other forces. Once we acknowledge that some patients want – and receive – inappropriate prescription medication (Linder and Stafford 2001), and that some even request such pharmaceutical souvenirs for their children, we are on the way to a form of understanding that will help to guide us in applying and even disseminating the best available evidence and cases, some of them unrelated to the one we started with.

There is another lesson that runs, albeit tacitly, through our cases. It actually affects all of health care, as well as debates over evidence, best practice, and policy. It is that many people are just ignorant about how the world, including the world of human biology, is put together and how it works. We actually know a great deal in the realm of clinical practice. We know, for instance, that antibiotics do not cure viral infections. This in turn calls for some sort of explanation as to why so many people request antibiotics for their viral infections – together with explanations as to why there is such great public demand for other interventions, remedies, therapies, unguents, lotions, and potions for which evidence is lacking.

We may fault education systems or the news media or even clinicians themselves, but the unhappy fact is that the growth of evidence-based practice has occurred in parallel with a burgeoning of interest in, and demand for, interventions for which either the evidence is weak or for which there is no evidence at all. Policy makers have as constituents people who live in both camps. Strikingly, what both groups – the scientists and the mystics – have in common is that neither has adequate tolerance for ambiguity and uncertainty.

Evidence-based genetics

Completion of the effort to sequence the human genome, announced in February 2001, will have, among its many effects, a reshuffling of research priorities and the creation of great challenges in clinical practice, public policy, and the lives of many ordinary people. Moreover, what was already a probabilistic science was rendered all the more complex when, in consequence of the milestone in identifying human genetic structure, estimates of the number of human genes were reduced as much as four- and five-fold, to about 30 000. This has already caused a shift in attention, and research, from structural genetics to functional genetics and a commensurate increase in complexity: There are just as many functions to explain as ever, but fewer structures to do it with.

A discussion of genetics is appropriate in the context of public health, public policy, and indeterminacy for a number of reasons:

- Genetics will turn out to be a primary engine in our understanding of population-based prevention and care (Khoury, Burke, and Thomson 2000).
- Genetics poses fundamental challenges for policy makers grappling with health benefits, discrimination, communication, and stigma (Annas and Elias 1992).
- Genetic information is complex and individual genes do not stand in an isomorphic relation to the proteins they express; gene expression profile analysis will have extraordinary consequences for our understanding of disease (King and Sinha 2001).

What is more, every issue, problem, and challenge we have dealt with so far – from the conceptual foundations of evidence-based practice and the research synthesis revolution to meta-evidence, data mining, and bedside decision making – will re-emerge and require re-evaluation under a genetic lamp.

Genetic evidence, or what we have learned from individual studies and systematic reviews, is accreting at an extraordinary rate, and yet it will be applied by clinicians who, in many cases, never became comfortable with research synthesis in the first place. In fact, though, "systematic genomics" may provide the kind of analytical traction needed to make sense finally of subgroup variation in all human subjects research, either at the level of the clinical trial or at the level of the systematic review. Understanding of such subgroup variations will be essential for future clinical decision making.

Here is an example. A review that included 18 of 333 drug reaction studies and 22 of 61 variant allele studies concludes that:

The emergence of pharmacogenomics may herald a new era of individualized therapy. Hence, nonpreventable [adverse drug reactions (ADR)] may become at least in part preventable, as a first step in optimizing drug therapy with genetic information. This study provides empirical evidence that the use of pharmacogenomics could potentially reduce ADRs, a problem of major significance . . . In the future, we may all carry a "gene chip assay report" that contains our unique genetic profile that would be consulted before drugs are prescribed. However, the application of pharmacogenomics information faces significant challenges, and further basic science, clinical and policy research is needed to determine in what areas pharmacogenomics can have the greatest impact, how it can be incorporated into practice, and what are its societal implications. (Phillips et al. 2001: 2277–8)

This augurs a new and potentially perilous course in evidence-based practice and policy, as we now need to make inferences from probabilistic data and systematic reviews in support of decisions that, as well as affecting life and death, will affect how we think of ourselves and the kinds of stances we should take regarding disease and health interventions.

The future of human subjects research

Consider the breadth of research into the genetic causes of disease and the best treatments or drugs for managing those diseases:

We now have reason to believe that different groups of genes are expressed by breast cancers with *BRCA1* and *BRCA2* mutations and that "a heritable mutation influences the gene-expression profile of the cancer" (Hedenfalk et al. 2001), and that tamoxifen reduces breast cancer incidence among healthy *BRCA2* carriers (King et al. 2001). Now, wouldn't it be interesting if we had data about genetic variations that influence, say, susceptibility to environmental tobacco smoke (or *any* environmental toxin)? The utility of screening mammograms? Otitis media response to antibiotics? Or how would you like further genetic subgroup analyses bearing on the questions of other diseases' response to other drugs, to susceptibility, to survivability, etc., etc? The information could inform everything from recommendations for counseling and prophylactic surgery (Huntsman et al. 2001), to the communication of good news (Gryfe et al. 2000).

In cardiology – domain for some of the most exciting and controversial work in systematic science and research synthesis – we are learning of connections or links between increased or decreased risk of heart attacks and tissue plasminogen activator gene polymorphisms (van der Bom et al. 1997), factor VII gene polymorphisms (Iacoviello et al. 1998), and polymorphisms for a gene that alters the rate of alcohol metabolism, leading to breathless news reports about the potentially beneficial effects of moderate alcohol consumption (Hines et al. 2001).

This is just a small taste of a vast new research program, a program that is in its infancy but which promises transformations as great as any in the history of the health sciences. Linkages or, rather, the absence of linkages between old systematic science and new, genome-based, systematic science, will have a remarkable – no, a *phenomenal* – consequence for research and practice: For this new science to be applied completely and appropriately, all our studies of all our maladies must be re-done to take into account genetic information. Pick the most contentious meta-analyses you want and imagine what it would be like to do them all over again, but with comprehensive genomic data included.

Great excitement attaches to the new genetics and pharmacogenomics, and with good reason. What remains to be seen is whether this science will reduce or increase uncertainty, and if so, in what areas. It might, for instance, be the case that we will acquire greater clinical confidence at the price of lesser confidence in ethical, social, or policy realms. This means that we need to devote increasingly greater resources to addressing challenges in these realms. We need to provide some guidance here, starting in the next section and continuing in Chapter 7.

Uncertainty and policy, revisited

The president of Britain's Royal Society, in an anniversary address, actually celebrated the role of uncertainty in policy: "I believe the admittedly awkward costs of wide and open consultation, and of open admission of uncertainty, are outweighed by their trust-promoting benefits. This is, let us not forget, exactly the recipe followed by science – open and free contest in the marketplace of ideas. It is a recipe that has served us well" (Lord May 2001). What this can teach us is that the long view, sometimes the very long view, can actually optimize policy based on shared values. It will not reduce the tension between the need to act and the brute fact of uncertainty, but it can help us see our way clear to recognizing that as long as uncertainty is an unavoidable feature of the decision-making landscape, then no decision can be evaluated without some wiggle room to accommodate error.

The demand for more research, aimed at reducing uncertainty as much as possible, may be tempered by the realization that, in any case, "Research rarely provides information that would have an immediate effect on a pending decision. Rather it provides background knowledge that changes understanding and might influence later deliberations, not only about a policy or program that has been evaluated but about others as well" (Cook et al. 1992: 334). This is not to say that there is research that should or may not be performed – it would on any theory of morality constitute scientific or political negligence to fail to *try* to answer our most pressing questions. But for those domains in which we have not gotten around to the science yet, or in those in which it would not matter, or even in those in which science has nothing to say, then our task is to do our best with the data – the messy, conflicted, and controversial data – at hand. It is a case for policy makers in which they must play with the cards they have been dealt:

It is, however, not enough for Government to be getting the right advice from the most informed people, and taking the right actions on that basis. Although, of course, such right advice and action must surely underlie all else, it is also important that the process be sufficiently open and inclusive that it engenders public confidence and democratic assent. For the Royal Society, one implication is that the usefulness of our advice, in the eyes both of policy-makers and of the wider public, depends on getting the science right (which, for all its difficulties, for us is the easy bit, where we have real authority), but also on getting our processes right.[3] (Lord May 2001)

In other words, good process will produce good policy more often than otherwise. Well, what does good science policy process look at when considering systematic reviews of important health issues? Surely we do not want it to have the look and feel of, say, the process that accompanies screening mammography. And, as ever, it will have to be recognized as fallible. You just do the best you can. A solid and quite useful introduction to, and review of, the use of research synthesis in public health policy suggests that a good way to begin is by "Adopting a neutral starting point, giving fair consideration to all relevant data, giving interest groups a chance to bring data to the committee for consideration, and avoiding bias and conflict of interest in the choice of committee members" (Stoto 2000: 354).

We also have a nontrivial, if checkered, track record to appeal to. It is not as if we are starting *ab initio* in trying to figure out how best to infer from science to policy, although systematic genetics will doubtless provide excellent challenges:

Synthesis of research findings has a long-standing tradition in science. While synthesis is currently required in the US food and drug regulatory process, formal meta-analysis may substitute for a pivotal study or broaden the generalizability of drug efficacy through a preplanned meta-analysis. Preplanned meta-analysis of individual trials with deliberately introduced heterogeneity may maximize the generalizability of results from randomized trials. Combining observational data may help to support an alternative claim or to quantify adverse events. In this setting, methods to address potentially greater sources of bias are required. Overall, meta-analysis adds evidence through the synthesis study findings and permits examination of how treatment effects vary across subgroups, such as age and sex, and across study settings. (Berlin and Colditz 1999: 830)

We need to appeal to this track record for a number of reasons. It provides perspective. It provides data. We need the data for policy not because one more bit will push over some epistemological edge and help achieve closure but in support of a "reliable method for comparing and contrasting the effectiveness of interventions in achieving health outcomes" to help sort out priorities and to inform our values (Woolf 1999).

It is often said that science is value laden. What is in part intended by this is that science is stuck in a conceptual trap or mire such that objectivity and neutrality are impossible. I think this view is mistaken, and that not only can we identify our values, we can evaluate them in environments where we are not beholden to them. We can re-evaluate the things we value, and, indeed, must do so. This has in the past helped us to improve our values. In the same way that scientific progress was held to be progressive, it could be that policy and values will be too, and that systematic science might help lead the way.

NOTES

1 See Goodman and Prineas (1996) for a discussion of some curriculum development goals.
2 The authors of the *Lancet* articles are themselves contributors to the literature on the quality of Cochrane reviews (Olsen et al. 2001). Seekers of irony will appreciate that the first *Lancet* article appeared in an edition with an article and editorial on "Practice guidelines developed by specialty societies" (Grilli et al. 2000).
3 Lord May was chief scientific adviser to the British government between 1995 and 2000. His remarks continue and are worth hearing:

   This is why we are putting great effort into conducting all our studies openly and inclusively, allowing as much opportunity as practicable for interested parties to have input to the questions we should be asking. . . . More generally, these activities acknowledge that society needs to do a better job of asking what kind of tomorrow we create with the possibilities that science offers, subject to the constraints which science clarifies. Such decisions are governed by values, beliefs, feelings; science has no special voice in such democratic debates about values. But science does serve a crucial function in painting the landscape of facts and uncertainties against which such societal debates take place. (Lord May 2001)

7

Ethics and evidence

We are informed about everything. We know nothing.   Saul Bellow (1977)

Ethical issues raised by meta-analysis/systematic review/research synthesis constitute the threads that have run throughout the preceding chapters. In this chapter, the threads will be pulled together with the goal of identifying the obligations of clinicians firstly and then clinical investigators, research synthesizers, and review boards. The intersection of ethics and evidence is an instance of the problem of ethical decision making in contexts of scientific uncertainty. That said, an "ethical best practice" is proposed for dealing with the practical challenges raised by evidence-based medicine, showing that ethical practice is, in large part, scientifically sound practice.

Evidence-based practice and fallibility

We do research to try to find out how the world works. We can make an observation, conduct a test, perform an experiment. Then we note what happens. *All research is outcomes research.*

When we train a student or colleague how to do something, we appeal to history, to precedent, to what has worked, to what the books and sages say. *All training is about following guidelines.*

If the world were simpler, everything would fit together more tidily. Research would show us unambiguously whether a phenomenon existed, why a drug worked, if that glass of wine were a good idea in terms of cardiovascular health. And we'd get it right the first time – none of this back and forth, she-loves-me-she-loves-me-not biomedical research. *But the world is not simple.*

We therefore find ourselves in the following very interesting situation (it might or might not be a predicament): Our best efforts to learn about the world will often fail to give us the kind of closure we crave. This is partly because, contrary to our metaphors, our science is not like a puzzle, or if it is, the picture we are assembling is changing while we are assembling it. Neither is it like a bucket we try to fill up with facts; it is more like a smelter, constantly purifying or refining what we throw in. And it is certainly not like a book, such that we think of the question to which we want to know the answer, and then look it up. It is a situation not for the faint of heart, especially when it comes to human health and sickness and death. For all those cases in which we lack closure, there are still, nonetheless, human lives in the balance.

Yet be it a puzzle, a cauldron, or a book, medical science is not making things easy for us. This means that our uncertainty is not necessarily, or always, our fault. Try the following with friends, colleagues, or students: Begin counting off the series of integers "2, 4, 6, 8" – and then break off and ask for the series to be completed. With luck, they will proffer "10" as the next integer in the series, whereupon you correct them and say, "Actually, no, it's 11." Then, after a sufficiently awkward pause, you explain that the series of numbers you had in mind was one that increases three times by 2, and then three times by 3. So the series would actually be 2, 4, 6, 8, 11, 14, 17 . . . . Of course, now, even though they know your trick, they still do not know what comes next. The example is due to the philosopher Ludwig Wittgenstein, who famously asked, "How is it decided what is the right step to take at any particular stage?" (Wittgenstein 1968: 75e; cf. Goodman 1998e and especially Nelson 2000 for a nice account of what is at issue here with rule following, namely that there is always another possible rule to build on the previous one). One lesson is that the patterns we identify in science must, in principle, be open to revision.

What this means for us now is that there are many cases in evidence-based practice in which more evidence may reduce but will not eliminate uncertainty. This is of the greatest importance because it means that even at our best we will not know as much as we need to prevent, retard, or stop a harm from occurring. Earlier, in Chapters 1, 2, and 5, I asked versions of the following key questions:

- How should we make decisions in the face of scientific uncertainty?
- Under what circumstances, if any, is error morally blameworthy?
- How should the fallibility of our science affect judgments of blameworthiness?

The rest of this chapter will consist of an attempt to answer these questions in an arena illuminated more or less well by the light of systematic science.

Judgments under uncertainty and complexity

While there are many circumstances in which more information, more data, or more evidence will not solve one's problem or eliminate the uncertainty attaching to a decision, it does not follow that clinicians are absolved from having to learn some stuff in the first place. In fact, there is a great deal to learn, although we have done a generally poor job deciding what it is and how to learn or teach it. This has caused us to be held in the thrall of what has been called "the cult of information" (Horton 1999). Recall from Chapter 3 that evidence is information that we use in deciding whether to believe a statement or proposition. If, according to a bruised but standard model, what we mean by "knowledge" is a true belief that we hold because of good evidence, then mere or more information can serve mainly to gum up the works (cf. Cassell 1997).

Still, we need to adopt some sort of approach to uncertainty. I will suggest three stances: management, acknowledgment, and reduction.

First, uncertainty management. Part of the name of this section – "Judgments under uncertainty" – comes from the title of a fine, early article that assesses our reliance on rules of thumb when we are uncertain, and how bias can corrupt those heuristic principles (Tversky and Kahneman 1974). What this suggests is that we can begin to manage our uncertainty, in part by reducing or eliminating conceptual bias in decision making. "Bias" here means the kinds of cognitive inclinations we have to round off, cut corners, and retreat to conceptual laziness. One well-known example is the "misconception of chance," or the expectation "that a sequence of events generated by a random process will represent the essential characteristics of that process even when the sequence is short . . . Chance is commonly viewed as a self-correcting process . . ." (ibid: 1125). The best examples of this are in those confused beliefs about coin tossing, for instance that the sequence H-T-H-T-T-H is more likely than the sequence T-T-T-H-H-H because it seems more random. Similarly, our cognitive biases can lead us to impose patterns on data or sensory input such that we see faces on Mars, a man in the Moon, or Jesus in a burnt tortilla (Carroll 2001).

The second way to respond to uncertainty is to acknowledge it and even share it with patients, "especially as it relates to diagnosis and outcome" (Logan and Scott 1996). If uncertainty is an unavoidable part of clinical practice, then it becomes deceptive not to acknowledge it. This is not to suggest that clinicians should worry patients with doubts that they might not be able to parse, but rather to set aside the air of omniscience and, well, certainty, that too many clinicians affect. To speak with too much confidence about the kinds of issues raised by the case studies in Chapter 6, for instance, would be deceptive, not encouraging. There are interesting problems related to how information should be presented to patients, as well as how much "spin" is appropriate. I am not here so much interested in that important debate, but hope only to promote the idea that sharing uncertainty, like error disclosure, is healthy for the healer and honest toward the healed. Such an approach is also likely to improve the informed or valid consent process. Psychologists and decision theorists have long known that patient preferences are easily manipulated, in part by positive spin (McNeil et al. 1982; cf. Hoffrage et al. 2000). All such machinations can corrupt the consent process and require special justification.

The third way in which I want to suggest that we should respond to uncertainty is perhaps the most obvious. It should perhaps be the strongest – reduce it. My project here is not to celebrate uncertainty or complexity so as to provide moral covering fire for the harms of ignorance; it is to remind us that the evidence-based project is an honest attempt to come to terms with the great and embarrassing fact that much of what has passed for clinical expertise and knowledge was custom, tradition, intuition, and luck. That even our best evidence will never be complete or definitive is not in itself a reason to slack off. When I suggested in Chapter 6 that, in an empirically uncertain environment, decision evaluation required some "wiggle room to accommodate error," it was not with the intent of excusing errors that could have been prevented.

Having turned a cold shoulder to the hoary notion of the intuitive "art of medicine," it might be the case that "clinical judgment" can now far more productively be seen as that critical faculty that is brought to bear when faced with uncertainty. We should neither wallow in it nor hope to overcome it. Rather, reducing conceptual biases, disclosure, and increased and improved learning are what we should consider as the core faculties that are enlisted when we perform this "clinical judgment." This has a wonderful advantage over other vague formulations or hopeful stipulations: It provides grounds for explaining the good outcomes on those occasions when we get it right.

Bounded rationality

The economist, philosopher, and computer scientist Herbert A. Sin (1916–2001) is perhaps best known for development of the concept of "bounded rationality," which, it seems to me, provides a useful complement to our three-fold approach to uncertainty. Simon was trying in part to establish a foundation for rational choice in an environment in which the decision maker is limited by knowledge and "computational capacity." We are just not smart enough to make completely rational decisions. (Keep in mind that the modern clinician does not lack information; it is not data ignorance that he or she faces, but ignorance at the larger level, the level at which one decides not to provide a smoking section, or to screen for breast cancer, or to prescribe an antibiotic for an ear infection.)

Simon's response to this state of affairs was to try to preserve rationality by circumscribing the domain in which it could apply. It followed that decision makers have to do as our policy makers did in Chapter 6, that is play with the cards they are dealt, make the best of a bad thing, choose the option that is, in essence, good enough:

A decision maker who chooses the best available alternative according to some criterion is said to optimize; one who chooses an alternative that meets or exceeds specified criteria, but that is not guaranteed to be either unique or in any sense the best, is said to satisfice . . . Faced with a choice situation where it is impossible to optimize, or where the computational cost of doing so seems burdensome, the decision maker may look for a satisfactory, rather than an optimal, alternative. Frequently, a course of action satisfying a number of constraints, even a sizeable number, is far easier to discover than a course of action maximizing some function. (Simon 1997a: 295; cf. Simon 1997b, 1999)

One reason to embrace such a view is that it rescues us from the extremes of decisional incapacity or inertia on the one side, and winging it on the other. This can be very helpful for those occasions in which "watchful waiting" is unacceptable and in which a decision needs to be made.

Here is an opportunity to remind ourselves that the class of cases here, while quite large, lives under the same conceptual roof as the numerous occasions on which ordinary clinicians make optimized decisions, and get it just right. The point of evidence-based practice and of outcomes research is to identify those decisions that are on target, so we can learn from them and share them. There are times when one fears that some of the objections to evidence-based practice are offered in the mistaken impression that it is

...ow suggesting that most clinicians are just not *...ing* it right. (Make ...istake – it can be the case that many physicia... *...r* their decisions are ...or without it being the case that *most* are... "Th... plain fact is that many ...ecisions made by physicians appear to be arbit...*ry* – highly variable, with no obvious explanation" and that this can co...*tute* "suboptimal or even harmful" care (Eddy 1990a).)

I want to say that ignorance reduction *j...* moral imperative (cf. Smith 1992). But this works only if ignorance re...*action* will improve health care; we are betting with evidence-based me...*icine* that it will. Further, if this is right, it puts to rout those arguments *...olding* that the "ascendancy of out-comes research is as much political *...* scientific" (Tanenbaum 1994).

Decision analysis

One way to try to make better clinical decisions is to adopt the tools of deci-sion analysis, a formal technique that incorporates the probabilities of clin-ical outcomes and the utility or value that patients place on the outcome. As is often advocated, a clinician and patient would work together to calculate the best decision, given the available options. This is thought to maximize both the consent process and patient autonomy and so is hailed as a power-ful tool for improved clinical ethics (Dowie 1994; Ubel and Lowenstein 1997; Elwyn et al. 2001; some of this position draws on important early work by Charles Culver and Bernard Gert (1982)).

Decision analysis requires discovery or assignment of values to the prob-ability of a clinical outcome (often death, pain, disability, or their opposites) and to the outcome's utility to the patient. We have some experience with the debate over the former: Everything that is right and wrong with clinical trials, outcomes research, and research synthesis needs to be factored in to the accuracy of these probability estimates. The assignment of utility is at least as complicated, with no small debate attaching to efforts to quantify quality of life, as with quality adjusted life-years (Singer et al. 1995; Harris 1995).

We should say that anything that improves valid consent and the ration-ality of health care decision making is noteworthy and positive. But decision analysis is complex and its foundations are controversial; this counsels caution. For instance, much decision analysis is informed by the inferential strategies of the Rev. Thomas Bayes (1702–1761), a Presbyterian minister whose 48-page manuscript, "Essay towards solving a problem in the doctrine of chances," was published posthumously – and nearly two-and-a-half centuries later has re-emerged as one of the most important documents in the history of scientific inquiry. Bayes' Theorem is a guide for updating belief when given new evidence; there are a number of points of entry for clinicians (Gross 1999; Malakoff 1999). What is striking is that Rev. Bayes has come to lead a movement, a crusade even, and this seems to have led to a level of unanimity of belief and purpose that, while exciting, may be misguided.

For one thing, there have long been serious philosophical objections to Bayes' Theorem. One such is that theories of confirmation should be able to explain scientific reasoning and scientific judgments, but Bayes' Theorem is mainly an approach to personal learning (Glymour 1980). In any case, there is a large and rich debate here (Earman 1992) and it could be that it will eventually have a salutary effect. What we should hope, though, is that partisans and advocates of the dead minister's approach will tune into the debate. What needs to be acknowledged all around is that there is certainly no closure on the questions raised by Bayes' Theorem, and hence on those aspects of formal decision theory that rely on it.

Also, "There are major differences between the academically recommended quantitative methods and the direct method reportedly used by many practicing physicians" in appraising diagnostic test accuracy (Reid, Lane, and Feinstein 1998). Despite this use of "academic" (again) as a pejorative, it means for us that there might be social or medico-social impediments to widespread adoption of decision analysis.

There is a further point to be made about patient preferences, and it is this: Sometimes they just do not make any sense, and depending on who is paying for the care, treatment, or intervention, what seemed like a straightforward matter of patient self-determination becomes a silly waste of public resources.

Cost considerations and futility

Considerations of cost, or cost-effectiveness, go hand in hand with decision analysis and, indeed, with all of evidence-based practice. It will not do, as some try, to suggest that attention to cost of care is itself somehow unethical, as if worrying about wasting resources were somehow celebrating a craving for filthy lucre. Indeed, there is a sense in which failure to attend to evidence, outcomes, and quality is unethical in part because it is inattention to the question as to whether a procedure, treatment, or intervention is worth paying for. If something does not work, or does not work well and this is not disclosed, then performing such an intervention is a rip-off (cf. Frazier and Mosteller 1995).

What is usually meant, however, by objections to evidence being used to control costs is that it is inappropriate to withhold care or cut corners for the sake of maximizing corporate or personal profit. And of course it is. But cost can be an important variable, and data about cost is essential for policy makers who need to balance budgets against effectiveness. Consider the following example:

Patients with nonvalvular atrial fibrillation are at high risk of ischemic stroke. Ischemic stroke can be prevented using either warfarin or aspirin. The efficacy of warfarin in preventing ischemic stroke is higher than that of aspirin, but warfarin is more likely than aspirin to cause bleeding, sometimes fatal, and it is more expensive, especially when the cost of monitoring prothrombin time is considered . . . Gage et al. (1995) did a cost-effectiveness analysis comparing warfarin and aspirin for stroke prophylaxis in patients with nonvalvular atrial fibrillation. They showed that warfarin was preferred to aspirin in patients at high risk for stroke but that aspirin was preferred to warfarin in patients at low risk for stroke. In this example, the question posed is not whether to treat patients with nonvalvular atrial fibrillation, but how to treat them. (Petitti 2000: 29)

What follows from examples such as this is that it would be ethically problematic *not* to attend to cost in this way. Doing so does not imply or entail that one has abandoned patients, sold out to corporate healthmongers, or otherwise gone over to the dark side of the Force. There might even be occasions in which decisions about the care of individual patients might be guided by cost – I am thinking here of cases in which there is accord between patient and clinician and neither wants to commit to a course of action that would include aggressive management of a condition unlikely to improve. This bumps against the issue of clinical futility, a complex area albeit one in which the coolest heads counsel better communication to achieve clarity of clinical goals – not threats to discontinue care, say, because a particular patient's life is somehow not worth the cost.

Note further that it is a little unfair to assign to individual clinicians responsibility for solving collective health care allocation problems. Many purported dilemmas of clinical practice evaporate when societies and governments do their duties in terms of public health infrastructure and

References

Abbot, D. 1983. *Biographical Dictionary of Scientists – Chemists*. New York: Peter Bedrick Books.

Achinstein, P. 1978. Concepts of evidence. *Mind* **87**: 22–45. Reprinted in *The Concept of Evidence*, ed. P. Achinstein (1983), pp. 145–74. Oxford: Oxford University Press.

Adams, A.S., Soumerai, S.B., Lomas, J., and Ross-Degnan, D. 1999. Evidence of self-report bias in assessing adherence to guidelines. *International Journal for Quality in Health Care* **11**: 187–92.

Ad Hoc Working Group for Critical Appraisal of the Medical Literature. 1987. Academia and clinic: A proposal for more informative abstracts of clinical articles. *Annals of Internal Medicine* **106**: 598–604.

Agency for Healthcare Research and Quality. 2001a. Evidence-based Practice Centers. Available at http://www.ahcpr.gov/clinic/epc/

Agency for Healthcare Research and Quality. 2001b. National Guideline Clearinghouse. Available at http://www.guidelines.gov/

Agency for Healthcare Research and Quality. 2001c. Management of acute otitis media. Evidence Report/Technology Assessment: Number 15. Available at http://www.ahrq.gov/clinic/otitisum.htm

Altman, D.G. 1994. The scandal of poor medical research. *British Medical Journal* **308**: 283–4.

Altman, D.G., Schulz, K.F., Moher, D., et al. 2001. The revised CONSORT statement for reporting randomized trials: Explanation and elaboration. *Annals of Internal Medicine* **134**: 663–94.

Anderson, J.G., and Goodman, K.W. 2001. *Ethics and Informatics: A Case-Study Approach*. New York: Springer Verlag.

Anderson, R.E., Hill, R.B., and Key, C.R. 1989. The sensitivity and specificity of clinical diagnosis during five decades: toward an understanding of necessary fallibility. *Journal of the American Medical Association* **261**: 1610–17.

Annas, G.J., and Elias, S., eds. 1992. *Gene Mapping: Using Law and Ethics as Guides*. Oxford: Oxford University Press.

Antiplatelet Trialists' Collaboration. 1994. Collaborative overview of randomised trials of antiplatelet therapy. Prevention of death, myocardial infarction, and stroke by prolonged antiplatelet therapy in various categories of patients. *British Medical Journal* **308**: 81–106.

Appelbaum, P., Roth, L., Lidz, C., Benson, P., and Winslade, W. 1987. False hopes and best data: consent to research and the therapeutic misconception. *Hastings Center Report* **2**: 20–4.

ASSERT. 2001. *A Standard for the Scientific and Ethical Review of Trials.* Available at http://www.assert-statement.org/

Associated Press. 2000. Clinical trials database for patients goes online. *The New York Times,* National Edition, February 29, 2000, p. A4.

Badgett, R.G., O'Keefe, M., and Henderson, M.C. 1997. Using systematic reviews in clinical education. *Annals of Internal Medicine* **126**: 886–91.

Bailar, J.C. 1995. The practice of meta-analysis. *Journal of Clinical Epidemiology* **48**: 149–57.

Barnes, D.E., and Bero, L.A. 1998. Why review articles on the health effects of passive smoking reach different conclusions. *Journal of the American Medical Association* **279**: 1566–70.

Bausell, R.B., Li, Y.F., Gau, M.L., and Soeken, K.L. 1995. The growth of meta-analytic literature from 1980 to 1993. *Evaluation & the Health Professions* **18**: 238–51.

Baylis, F. 1989. Persons with moral expertise and moral experts. In *Clinical Ethics: Theory and Practice,* ed. B. Hoffmaster, B. Freedman and G. Fraser, pp. 89–99. Clifton, NJ: Humana Press.

Begg, C., Cho, M., Eastwood, S., et al. 1996. Improving the quality of reporting of randomized controlled trials: the CONSORT statement. *Journal of the American Medical Association* **276**: 637–9.

Belkin, G. 1997. The technocratic wish: making sense and finding power in the "managed" medical marketplace. *Journal of Health Politics, Policy and Law* **22**: 509–32.

Bellow, S. 1977. *To Jerusalem and Back: A Personal Account.* New York: Avon.

Benson, K., and Hartz, A.J. 2000. A comparison of observational studies and randomized, controlled trials. *New England Journal of Medicine* **342**: 1878–86.

Berg, M. 1997. Problems and promises of the protocol. *Social Science and Medicine* **44**: 1081–8.

Berlin, J.A., and Colditz, G.A. 1999. The role of meta-analysis in the regulatory process for foods, drugs, and devices. *Journal of the American Medical Association* **281**: 830–4.

Berlin, J.A., and Rennie, D. 1999. Measuring the quality of trials: The quality of quality scales. *Journal of the American Medical Association* **282**: 1083–4.

Bero, L., and Rennie, D. 1995. The Cochrane Collaboration: preparing, maintaining, and disseminating systematic reviews of the effects of health care. *Journal of the American Medical Association* **274**: 1935–8.

Birkmeyer, J.D., Sharp, S.M., Finlayson, S.R., Fisher, E.S., and Wennberg, J.E. 1998. Variation profiles of common surgical procedures. *Surgery* **124**: 917–23.

Black, N. 1999. High-quality clinical databases: breaking down barriers. *Lancet* 353: 1205–6.

Black, N. 2001. Evidence based policy: proceed with care. *British Medical Journal* 323: 275–8.

Blumenthal, D., Campbell, E.G., Anderson, M.S., Causino, N., and Louis, K.S. 1997. Withholding research results in academic life science: evidence from a national survey of faculty. *Journal of the American Medical Association* 277: 1224–8.

van der Bom, J.G., de Knijff, P., Haverkate, F., et al. 1997. Tissue plasminogen activator and risk of myocardial infarction. The Rotterdam Study. *Circulation* 95: 2623–7.

Booth, A., compiler 1999. What proportion of healthcare is evidence based? Resource Guide. Available at http://www.shef.ac.uk/~scharr/ir/percent.html.

Bosk, C.L. 1981. *Forgive & Remember: Managing Medical Failure.* Chicago: University of Chicago Press.

Boyle, P.J., and Callahan, D. 2000. Physicians' use of outcomes data: Moral conflicts and potential resolutions. In *Getting Doctors to Listen: Ethics and Outcomes Data in Context*, ed. P.J. Boyle. Hastings Center Studies in Ethics, pp. 3–20. Washington, DC: Georgetown University Press.

Brennan, T.A. 2000. The Institute of Medicine report on medical errors – could it do harm? *New England Journal of Medicine* 342: 1123–5.

British Medical Journal. 1998. Fifty years of randomised controlled trials (editorial). *British Medical Journal* 317: no page given.

Broad, W.J. 1981. The publishing game: getting more for less. *Science* 211: 1137–9.

Brossette, S.E., Sprague, A.P., Hardin, J.M., Waites, K.B., Jones, W.T., and Moser, S.A. 1998. Association rules and data mining in hospital infection control and public health surveillance. *Journal of the American Medical Informatics Association* 5: 373–81.

Buetow, S., and Kenealy, T. 2000. Evidence-based medicine: the need for a new definition. *Journal of Evaluation in Clinical Practice* 6: 85–92.

Buñuel Álvarez, J.C. 2001. Medicina basada en la evidencia: una nueva manera de ejercer la pediatría. *Anales Españoles de Pediatría* 55: 440–52.

Burch, R.W. 1974. Are there moral experts? *The Monist* 58: 646–58.

Bureau of National Affairs. 2001. Five Minnesota health plans agree to use same protocols in effort to improve care. *BMA's Health Plan & Provider Report* 7: 383–4 (March 21, 2001).

Byar, D.P. 1980. Why data bases should not replace randomized clinical trials. *Biometrics* 36: 337–42.

Bynum, W.F., and Wilson, J.C. 1992. Periodical knowledge: medical journals and their editors in nineteenth-century Britain. In *Medical Journals and Medical Knowledge: Historical Essays*, ed. W.F. Bynum, S. Lock and R. Porter, pp. 29–48. London: Routledge.

Bynum, W.F., Lock, S., and Porter, R., eds. 1992. *Medical Journals and Medical Knowledge: Historical Essays.* London: Routledge.

Cabana, M.D., Rand, C.S., Powe, N.R., et al. 1999. Why don't physicians follow clinical practice guidelines? A framework for improvement. *Journal of the American Medical Association* 282:1458–65.

Cairns, J.A., Theroux, P., Lewis, H.D., Ezekowitz, M., Meade, T.W., and Sutton, G.C. 1998. Antithrombotic agents in coronary artery disease. *Chest* 114: 611S-33S.

Calder, R. 1965. Tyranny of the expert. *The Philosophical Journal* 2: 1–9.

Campazzi, E.J., and Lee, D.A. 1997. The history of outcomes assessment: An embarrassment to the medical profession. In *Tools for the Task: The Role of Clinical Guidelines*, ed. J.E. Casanova, pp. 171–81. Tampa, Fla.: American College of Physician Executives.

Canadian Task Force on the Periodic Health Examination. 1979. The periodic health examination. *Canadian Medical Association Journal* 121: 1193–1254.

Caplan, A.L. 1989. Moral experts and moral expertise: Do either exist? In *Clinical Ethics: Theory and Practice*, ed. B. Hoffmaster, B. Freedman, and G. Fraser, pp. 59–87. Clifton, NJ: Humana Press.

Carroll, R.T. 2001. Pareidol. *The Skeptic's Dictionary*. Available at http://www.skeptic.com/pareidol.html.

Cassell, E.J. 1997. Why should doctors read medical books? *Annals of Internal Medicine* 127: 576–8.

Center for the Evaluative Clinical Sciences. 1999. *The Dartmouth Atlas of Health Care 1999*. Chicago: American Hospital Association.

Centers for Disease Control and Prevention. 2001. Vaccinia (smallpox) vaccine: recommendations of the Advisory Committee on Immunization Practices (ACIP). MMWR 50: 1–25.

Chalmers, I. 1990. Underreporting research is scientific misconduct. *Journal of the American Medical Association* 263: 1405–8.

Chalmers, I., and Altman, D. 1995. Foreword. In *Systematic Reviews*, ed. I. Chalmers and D. Altman, pp. vii–ix. London: BMJ Publishing Group.

Chalmers, I., and Grant, A. 2001. Evidence-based medicine: Salutary lessons from the Collaborative Eclampsia Trial. American College of Physicians – American Society for Internal Medicine Online. Available at http://www.acponline.org/journals/ebm/janfeb96/notebook.htm.

Chalmers, I., Dickersin, K., and Chalmers, T.C. 1992. Getting to grips with Archie Cochrane's agenda. *British Medical Journal* 305: 786–8.

Chalmers, T.C. 1991. Problems induced by meta-analyses. *Statistics in Medicine* 10: 971–80.

Chalmers, T.C., Frank, C.S., and Reitman, D. 1990. Minimizing the three stages of publication bias. *Journal of the American Medical Association* 263: 1392–5.

Chassin, M.R. 1998. Is health care ready for Six Sigma quality? *Milbank Quarterly* 76: 575–91.

Chubin, D.E. 1976. The conceptualization of scientific specialties. *The Sociological Quarterly* 17: 448–76.

Clancy, C.M., and Eisenberg, J.M. 1998. Outcomes research: measuring the end results of health care. *Science* **282**: 245–6.

Clark, R.W. 1971. *Einstein: The Life and Times.* New York: World Publishing.

Clark, H.D., Wells, G.A., Huët, C., et al. 1999. Assessing the quality of randomized trials: reliability of the Jadad scale. *Controlled Clinical Trials* **20**: 448–52.

Clarke, M., and Oxman, A.D., eds. 2001. *Cochrane Reviewers' Handbook 4.1.4* [updated October 2001]. The Cochrane Library, Issue 4, 2001 (Updated quarterly). Oxford: Update Software.

Cochrane, A.L. 1972. *Effectiveness and Efficiency: Random Reflections on Health Services.* London: Nuffield Provincial Hospitals Trust (reprinted 1989, Royal Society of Medicine Press, London).

Cochrane, A.L. 1979. 1931–1971: a critical review, with particular reference to the medical profession. In *Medicines for the Year 2000.* London: Office of Health Economics, 1979, pp. 1–11. Available at http://www.cochrane.org/cochrane/cc-broch.htm#R2.

Cochrane Collaboration. 2001. Cochrane brochure. Available at http://www.cochrane.org/cochrane/cc-broch.htm#PRINCIPLES.

Cohen, S.J., Weinberger, M., Hui, S.L., Tierney, W.M., and McDonald, C.J. 1985. The impact of reading on physicians' nonadherence to recommended standards of medical care. *Social Science and Medicine* **21**: 909–14.

Colditz, G., Glasziou, P., and Irwig, L. 2001. *Systematic Reviews in Health Care: A Practical Guide.* Cambridge: Cambridge University Press.

Committee on Quality of Health Care in America, Institute of Medicine. 2001. *Crossing the Quality Chasm: A New Health System for the 21st Century.* Washington, DC: National Academy Press.

Concato, J., Shah, N., and Horwitz, R.I. 2000. Randomized, controlled trials, observational studies, and the hierarchy of research designs. *New England Journal of Medicine* **342**: 1887–92.

Cook, D.J., Greengold, N.L., Ellrodt, A.G., and Weingarten, S.R. 1997. The relation between systematic reviews and practice guidelines. *Annals of Internal Medicine* **127**: 210–16.

Cook, D.J., Mulrow, C.D., and Haynes, B. 1998. Synthesis of best evidence for clinical decisions. In *Systematic Reviews: Synthesis of Best Evidence for Health Care Decisions,* ed. C. Mulrow and D. Cook, pp. 5–12. Philadelphia: American College of Physicians.

Cook, D.J., Sackett, D.L., and Spitzer, W.O. 1995. Methodologic guidelines for systematic reviews of randomized control trials in health care from the Potsdam consultation on meta-analysis. *Journal of Clinical Epidemiology* **48**:167–71.

Cook, T.D., Cooper, H., Cordray, D.S., et al. 1992. *Meta-Analysis for Explanation: A Casebook.* New York: Russell Sage Foundation.

Cooper, H., and Hedges, L.V., eds. 1994. *The Handbook of Research Synthesis.* New York: Russell Sage Foundation.

Costa-Bouzas, J., Takkouche, B., Caradso-Suárez, and C., Spiegelman, D. 2001. HEpiMA: software for the identification of heterogeneity in meta-analysis. *Computer Methods and Programs in Biomedicine* **64**: 101–7.

Coughlin, S. and Beauchamp, T., eds. 1996. *Ethics and Epidemiology*. Oxford: Oxford University Press.

Coughlin, S., Soskolne, C., and Goodman, K. 1977. *Case Studies in Public Health Ethics*. Washington, DC: American Public Health Association.

Culotta, E. 1993. Study: male scientists publish more, women cited more. *The Scientist* July 26, **7**: 14–15.

Culpeper, N., Cole, A., and Rowland, W. 1678. The Practice of Physick, in seventeen several books: *Wherein is plainly set forth, The Nature, Cause, Differences, and Several sorts of Signs, Together with the Cure of all Diseases in the Body . . . Being chiefly a Translation of The Works of that Learned and Renowned Doctor, Lazarus Riverius, Sometimes Councellor and Physician to the King of France: To which are added Four Books containing Five hundred and thirteen Observations of Famous Cures.* London: George Sawbridge. (The cure quoted is titled "The Pestilence" and is the 452nd observation in the "*History of Famous and Rare Cures &c.*")

Culpepper, L., and Froom, J. 1995. Otitis media with effusion in young children: treatment in search of a problem. *Journal of the American Board of Family Practice* **8**: 1–12.

Culver, C.M., and Gert, B. 1982. *Philosophy in Medicine: Conceptual and Ethical Problems in Medicine and Psychiatry*. Oxford: Oxford University Press.

DARPA. 2001. Bio-Surveillance System, Proposer Information Pamphlet (Broad Agency Announcement [BAA] #01–17). Available at http://www.darpa.mil/ito/Solicitations.html.

Davidoff, F., DeAngelis, C.D., Drazen, J.M., et al. 2001. Sponsorship, authorship, and accountability. *New England Journal of Medicine* **345**: 825–6.

Davidoff, F., Haynes, B., Sackett, D., and Smith, R. 1995. Evidence-based medicine; a new journal to help doctors identify the information they need. *British Medical Journal* **310**: 1085–6.

Dayton, C.S., Ferguson, J.S., Hornick, D.B., and Peterson, M.W. 2000. Evaluation of an Internet-based decision-support system for applying the ATS/CDC guidelines for tuberculosis preventive therapy. *Medical Decision Making* **20**: 1–6.

de Clercq, P.A., Hasman, A., Blom, J.A., and Korsten, H.H.M. 2001. Design and implementation of a framework to support the development of clinical guidelines. *International Journal of Medical Informatics* **64**: 285–318.

Department of Veterans Affairs. 2001. New choices in cancer care for veterans. Available at http://www.va.gov/cancer/page.cfm?pg=9.

Dickersin, K. 1990. The existence of publication bias and risk factors for its occurrence. *Journal of the American Medical Association* **263**: 1385–9.

Dickersin, K., and Min, Y.I. 1993a. Publication bias: the problem that won't go away. *Annals of the New York Academy of Sciences*, **703**: 135–46.

Dickersin, K., and Min, Y.I. 1993b. NIH clinical trials and publication bias. *Online Journal of Current Clinical Trials,* April 28: Document No. 50.

Dickersin, K., Chan, S., Chalmers, T.C., Sacks, H.S., and Smith, H. 1987. Publication bias and clinical trials. *Controlled Clinical Trials* 8: 343–53.

Dickersin, K., Min, Y.-I., and Meinert, C.L. 1992. Factors influencing publication of research results: follow-up of applications submitted to two institutional review boards. *Journal of the American Medical Association* 267: 374–8.

Diemente, D., and Campbell, R. 1983. Sir Humphrey Davy (1778–1829). Woodrow Wilson Leadership Program in Chemistry website. Available at http://www.woodrow.org/ teachers/ci/1992/Davy.html.

Doddi, S., Marathe, A., Ravi, S.S., and Torney, D.C. 2001. Discovery of association rules in medical data. *Medical Informatics & The Internet in Medicine* 26: 25–33.

Donabedian, A. 1980. *The Definition of Quality and Approaches to its Assessment,* Vol. 1. Chicago: Health Administration Press.

Dowie, J. 1994. Decision analysis: the ethical approach to medical decision-making. In *Principles of Health Care Ethics,* ed. R. Gillon, pp. 412–34. Chichester: John Wiley.

Duhem, P. 1962. *The Aim and Structure of Physical Theory,* transl. P.P. Wiener. New York: Atheneum (originally published in 1954 by Princeton University Press).

Durieux, P., Nizard, R., Ravaud, P., Mounier, N., and Lepage, E. 2000. A clinical decision support system for prevention of venous thromboembolism: Effect on physician behavior. *Journal of the American Medical Association* 283: 2816–21.

Earman, J. 1992. *Bayes or Bust? A Critical Examination of Bayesian Confirmation Theory.* Cambridge, Mass.: The MIT Press.

Easterbrook, P.J., Berlin, J.A., Gopalan, R., and Matthews, D.R. 1991. Publication bias in clinical research. *Lancet* 337: 867–72.

Eddy, D.M. 1990a. Clinical decision making: from theory to practice. The challenge. *Journal of the American Medical Association* 263: 287–90.

Eddy, D.M. 1990b. Clinical decision making: from theory to practice. Practice policies – guidelines for methods. *Journal of the American Medical Association* 263: 1839–41.

Eddy, D.M. 1991. Clinical decision making: from theory to practice. The individual vs society. Resolving the conflict. *Journal of the American Medical Association* 265: 2399–401, 2405–6.

Eddy, D.M. 1993. Three battles to watch in the 1990s. *Journal of the American Medical Association* 270: 520–6.

Eddy, D.M., and Billings, J. 1988. The quality of medical evidence: implications for quality of care. *Health Affairs* Spring, 7: 19–32.

Eisenberg, J.M. 2001. What does evidence mean? Can the law and medicine be reconciled? *Journal of Health Politics, Policy and Law* 26: 369–81.

Elwyn, G., Edwards, A., Eccles, M., and Rovner, D. 2001. Decision analysis in patient care. *Lancet* 358: 571–4.

Emparanza Knörr, J.I. 2001. Medicina basada en la evidencia: un aprendizaje imprescindible. *Anales Españoles de Pediatría* 55: 397–9.

Engelhardt, H.T., and Caplan, A.L., eds. 1987. *Scientific Controversies: Case Studies in the Resolution and Closure of Disputes in Science and Technology.* Cambridge: Cambridge University Press.

Environmental Health Information Service. 2001. Ninth Report on Carcinogens. US Department of Health and Human Services, National Toxicology Program. Available at http://www.ehis.niehs.nih.gov/roc.

Environmental Protection Agency. 1992. *Respiratory Health Effects of Passive Smoking: Lung Cancer and Other Disorders.* Washington, D.C.: Government Printing Office (EPA/600/6–90/006F; GPO: 0555–000–00407–2).

Erwin, E. 1984. Establishing causal connections: meta-analysis and psychotherapy. *Midwest Studies in Philosophy* 9: 421–36.

Erwin, E., and Siegel, H. 1989. Is confirmation differential? *British Journal for the Philosophy of Science* 40: 105–19.

Evans, J.T., Nadjari, H.I., and Burchell, S. 1990. Quotational and reference accuracy in surgical journals. *Journal of the American Medical Association* 263: 1353–4.

Evidence-based Medicine Working Group. 1992. Evidence-based medicine: a new approach to teaching the practice of medicine. *Journal of the American Medical Association* 268: 2420–5.

Eysenck, H.J. 1978. An exercise in mega-silliness. *American Psychologist* 33: 517.

Feinstein, A.R. 1992. Critique of review article, "Environmental tobacco smoke: Current assessment and future directions." *Toxicologic Pathology* 20: 303–5.

Feinstein, A.R. 1995. Meta-analysis: statistical alchemy for the 21st century. *Journal of Clinical Epidemiology* 48: 71–9.

Feinstein, A.R. 1996. Meta-analysis and meta-analytic monitoring of clinical trials. *Statistics in Medicine* 15: 1273–80.

Feinstein, A.R., and Esdaile, J.M. 1987. Incidence, prevalence, and evidence: scientific problems in epidemiologic statistics for the occurrence of cancer. *American Journal of Medicine* 82: 113–23.

Feinstein, A.R., and Horwitz, R.I. 1997. Problems in the "evidence" of "evidence-based medicine." *American Journal of Medicine* 103: 529–35.

Ferguson, J.H. 1997. Interpreting scientific evidence: comparing the National Institutes of Health Consensus Development Program and courts of law. *The Judges' Journal* Summer, 36: 21–4, 83–4.

Feyerabend, P. 1975. *Against Method.* London: Verso.

Feyerabend, P. 1978. *Science in a Free Society.* London: Verso.

Field, M.J., and Lohr, K.N., eds. 1990. *Clinical Practice Guidelines: Directions for a New Program.* Institute of Medicine. Washington, DC: National Academy Press.

Field, M.J., and Lohr, K.N., eds. 1992. *Guidelines for Clinical Practice: From Development to Use.* Institute of Medicine. Washington, DC: National Academy Press.

Finder, J.M. 2000. The future of practice guidelines: should they constitute conclusive evidence of the standard of care? *Health Matrix: Journal of Law-Medicine* 10: 67–117.

Flores, G., Lee, M., Bauchner, H., and Kastner, B. 2000. Pediatricians' attitudes, beliefs, and practices regarding clinical practice guidelines: a national survey. *Pediatrics* 105(3 Pt 1): 496–501.

Foster, K.R., and Huber, P.W. 1999. *Judging Science: Scientific Knowledge and the Federal Courts.* Cambridge, Mass.: The MIT Press.

Frank, P. 1949. Einstein's philosophy of science. *Reviews of Modern Physics* 21: 349–55.

Frazier, H.S., and Mosteller, F., eds. 1995. *Medicine Worth Paying For: Assessing Medical Innovations.* Cambridge, Mass.: Harvard University Press.

Freemantle, N., Eccles, M., Wood, J., et al. 1999. A randomized trial of evidence-based outreach (EBOR): rationale and design. *Controlled Clinical Trials* 20: 479–92.

Freudenheim, M. 2001a. Minnesota health plans to standardize treatments. *The New York Times*, National Edition, March 13, pp. C1, C9.

Freudenheim, M. 2001b. Florida employers will offer incentives to doctors. *The New York Times*, National Edition, November 16, p. C5.

Friedenwald, H. 1917. Oath and prayer of Maimonides. *Bulletin of the Johns Hopkins Hospital* 28: 260–1.

Gage, B.F., Cardinalli, A.B., Albers, G.W., and Owens, P.K. 1995. Cost-effectiveness of warfarin and aspirin for prophylaxis of stroke in patients with nonvalvular atrial fibrillation. *Journal of the American Medical Association* 274: 1839–45.

Galal, G., Cook, D.J., and Holder, L.B. 1997. Improving scalability in a knowledge discovery system by exploiting parallelism. In *Proceedings of the Third International Conference on Knowledge Discovery and Data Mining*, ed. D. Heckerman, H. Mannila, D. Pregibon, and R. Uthurusamy, pp. 171–4. Menlo Park, Calif.: American Association of Artificial Intelligence.

Garfield, E. 1979. *Citation Indexing – Its Theory and Application in Science, Technology, and Humanities.* New York: John Wiley & Sons.

Garfunkel, J.M., Ulshen, M.H., Hamrick, H.J., and Lawson, E.E. 1990. Problems identified by secondary review of accepted manuscripts. *Journal of the American Medical Association* 263: 1369–71.

Garnick, D.W., Hendricks, A.M., and Brennan, T.A. 1991. Can practice guidelines reduce the number and costs of malpractice claims? *Journal of the American Medical Association* 266: 2856–60.

Gatens-Robinson, E. 1986. Clinical judgment and the rationality of the human sciences. *Journal of Medicine and Philosophy* 11(2): 167–78.

Gawande, A. 1999. The cancer-cluster myth. *The New Yorker*, February 8: 34–7.

Gert, B. 1998. *Morality: Its Nature and Justification.* Oxford: Oxford University Press.

Giacomini, M.K., and Cook, D.J. 2000. Users' guides to the medical literature: XXIII. Qualitative research in health care: B. What are the results and how do they help me care for my patients? *Journal of the American Medical Association* 284: 478–82.

Gifford, D.R., Holloway, R.G., Frankel, M.R., et al. 1999. Improving adherence to dementia guidelines through education and opinion leaders: a randomized, controlled trial. *Annals of Internal Medicine* **131**: 237–46.

Gilovich, T., Vallone, R., and Tversky, A. (1985). The hot hand in basketball: on the misperception of random sequences. *Cognitive Psychology* **17**: 295–314.

Glass, G.V. 1976. Primary, secondary, and meta-analysis of research. *Educational Researcher* **6**: 3–8.

Glass, G., and Kliegl, R. 1983. An apology for research integration in the study of psychotherapy. *Journal of Consulting and Clinical Psychology* **51**: 28–41.

Glass, G.V., McGaw, B., and Smith, M.L. 1981. *Meta-Analysis in Social Research.* Newbury Park, Calif.: Sage Publications.

Glymour, C. 1980. *Theory and Evidence.* Princeton, NJ: Princeton University Press.

González de Dios, J. 2001. De la medicina basada en la evidencia a la evidencia basada en la medicina. *Anales Expañoles de Pediatría* **55**: 429–39.

Good, P. 2001. *Resampling Methods: A Practical Guide to Data Analysis,* 2nd edn. Boston: Birkhauser.

Goodman, K.W. 1996. Codes of ethics in occupational and environmental health. *Journal of Occupational and Environmental Medicine* **38**: 882–3.

Goodman, K.W., ed. 1998a. *Ethics, Computing and Medicine: Informatics and the Transformation of Health Care.* New York: Cambridge University Press.

Goodman, K.W. 1998b. Meta-analysis: conceptual, ethical and policy issues. In *Ethics, Computing and Medicine: Informatics and the Transformation of Health Care,* ed. K.W. Goodman, pp. 139–67. Cambridge and New York: Cambridge University Press.

Goodman, K.W. 1998c. Ethical challenges. In *International Occupational and Environmental Medicine,* ed. J.A. Herzstein et al., pp. 86–96. St. Louis: Mosby.

Goodman, K.W. 1998d. Ethical and legal issues in use of decision support systems. In *Decision Support Systems,* ed. E. Berner, pp. 217–33. New York: Springer Verlag.

Goodman, K.W. 1998e. Outcomes, futility and health policy research. In *Ethics, Computing and Medicine: Informatics and the Transformation of Health Care,* ed. K.W. Goodman, pp. 116–38. Cambridge and New York: Cambridge University Press.

Goodman, K.W. 2000. Using the Web as a research tool. *MD Computing* **17**(5): 13–14.

Goodman, K.W., and Frumkin, H. 1997. Ethical issues in international occupational health. In *International Occupational and Environmental Medicine,* ed. L.E. Fleming, pp. 17–32. Beverly, Mass.: OEM Press.

Goodman, K.W., and Miller, R. 2001. Ethics and health informatics: users, standards and outcomes. In *Medical Informatics: Computer Applications in Health Care and Biomedicine,* ed. E.H. Shortliffe et al., pp. 257–81. New York: Springer-Verlag.

Goodman, K.W., and Prineas, R. 1996. Toward an ethics curriculum in epidemiology. In *Ethics and Epidemiology.* ed. S. Coughlin and T. Beauchamp, pp. 290–303. Oxford: Oxford University Press.

Gøtzsche, P.C., and Olsen, O. 2000. Is screening for breast cancer with mammography justifiable? *Lancet* **355**: 129–34.

Granata, A.V., and Hillman, A.L. 1998. Competing practice guidelines: using cost-effectiveness analysis to make optimal decisions. *Annals of Internal Medicine* **128**: 56–63.

Greenhalgh, T. 2000. *How to Read a Paper: The Basics of Evidence Based Medicine.* London: BMJ Publishing Group.

Grilli, R., Magrini, N., Penna, A., Mura, G., and Liberati, A. 2000. Practice guidelines developed by specialty societies: the need for a critical appraisal. *Lancet* **355**: 103–6.

Grimshaw, J.M., and Russell, I.T. 1993. Effect of clinical guidelines on medical practice: a systematic review of rigorous evaluations. *Lancet* **342**: 1317–22.

Gross, R. 1999. *Making Medical Decisions.* Philadelphia: American College of Physicians.

Gryfe, R., Kim, H., Hsieh, E.T., et al. 2000. Tumor microsatellite instability and clinical outcome in young patients with colorectal cancer. *New England Journal of Medicine* **342**: 69–77.

Guyatt, G., and Rennie, D., eds. 2001. *User's Guide to the Medical Literature: Essentials of Evidence-Based Clinical Practice.* Chicago: AMA Press.

Haack, S. 2001. An epistemologist in the bramble-bush: at the Supreme Court with Mr. Joiner. *Journal of Health Politics, Policy and Law* **26**: 217–48.

Ham, C., Hunter, D.J., and Robinson, R. 1995. Evidence based policymaking. *British Medical Journal* **310**: 71–2.

Hankins, G. 1987. The paradox of expertise. *Engineering Education* **77**: 302–5.

Hardwig, J. 1985. Epistemic dependence. *The Journal of Philosophy* **82**: 335–49.

Hardwig, J. 1991. The role of trust in knowledge. *The Journal of Philosophy* **88**: 693–708.

Harris, J. 1995. Double jeopardy and the veil of ignorance – a reply. *Journal of Medical Ethics* **21**: 151–7.

Haycox, A., Bagust, A., and Walley, T. 1999. Clinical guidelines – the hidden costs. *British Medical Journal* **318**: 391–3.

Haynes, R.B. 1991. How clinical journals could serve clinician readers better. In *The Future of Medical Journals,* ed. S. Lock, pp. 116–26. London: BMJ Publications.

Hayward, R.S.A., Wilson, M.C., Tunis, S.R., and Bass, E.B., for the Evidence-Based Medicine Working Group. 1995. Users' guides to the medical literature VIII: how to use clinical practice guidelines. A: are the recommendations valid? *Journal of the American Medical Association* **274**: 570–4.

Hayward, R.S.A., Wilson, M.C., Tunis, S.R., Bass, E.B., Rubin, H.R., and Haynes, R.B. 1993. More informative abstracts of articles describing clinical practice guidelines. *Annals of Internal Medicine* **118**: 731–7.

Hedenfalk, I., Duggan, D., Chen, Y., et al. 2001. Gene-expression profiles in hereditary breast cancer. *New England Journal of Medicine* **344**: 539–48.

Hedges, L.V., and Olkin, I. 1980. Vote counting methods in research synthesis. *Psychological Bulletin* **88**: 359–69.

Hedges, L.V., and Olkin, I. 1985. *Statistical Methods for Meta-Analysis*. San Diego: Academic Press.

Hill, A.B. 1971. *Principles of Medical Statistics*, 9th edn, London: Lancet.

Hines, L.M., Stampfer, M.J., Ma, J., et al. 2001. Genetic variation in alcohol dehydrogenase and the beneficial effect of moderate alcohol consumption on myocardial infarction. *New England Journal of Medicine* 344: 549–55.

Hippocrates. 1983. Prognosis. In *Hippocratic Writings*, ed. G.E.R. Lloyd, transl. J. Chadwisk and W.N. Mann, pp. 170–85. London: Penguin.

Hoffrage, U., Lindsey, S., Hertwig, R., and Gigerenzer, G. 2000. Communicating statistical information. *Science* 290: 2261–2.

Horton, R. 1999. The information wars. *Lancet* 353: 164–5.

Horton, R. 2001a. The clinical trial: deceitful, disputable, unbelievable, unhelpful, and shameful – what next? *Controlled Clinical Trials* 22: 593–604.

Horton, R. 2001b. Screening mammography – an overview revisited. *Lancet* 358:1284–5.

Horton, R., and Smith, R. 1999. Time to register randomised trials. *Lancet* 354: 1138–9. (version of Smith and Horton 1999).

Hume, D. 1739 (1969, 1985). *A Treatise of Human Nature*, ed. E.C. Mossner. Harmondsworth: Penguin.

Hunt, M. 1997. *How Science Takes Stock: The Story of Meta-Analysis*. New York: Russell Sage Foundation.

Hunter, J.E., and F.L. Schmidt. 1990. *Methods of Meta-Analysis: Correcting Error and Bias in Research Findings*. New York: Sage Publications.

Huntsman, D.G., Carneiro, F., Lewis, F.R., et al. 2001. Early gastric cancer in young, asymptomatic carriers of germ-line E-cadherin mutations. *New England Journal of Medicine* 344: 1904–9.

Hurwitz, B. 1999. Legal and political considerations of clinical practice guidelines. *British Medical Journal* 318: 661–4.

Huth, E.J. 1986. Irresponsible authorship and wasteful publication. *Annals of Internal Medicine* 104: 257–8.

Hyman, D.A., and Silver, C. 2001. Just what the patient ordered: the case for result-based compensation arrangements. *Journal of Law, Medicine & Ethics* 29: 170–3.

Iacoviello, L., Di Castelnuovo, A., de Knijff, P., et al. 1998. Polymorphisms in the coagulation factor VII gene and the risk of myocardial infarction. *New England Journal of Medicine* 338: 79–85.

Institute of Medicine. 2000. *Protecting Data Privacy in Health Services Research*. Washington, DC: National Academy Press.

International Committee of Medical Journal Editors. 1997. Uniform requirements for manuscripts submitted to biomedical journals. *Journal of the American Medical Association* 277: 927–34.

Ioannidis, J.P.A., Haidich, A.-B., Pappa, M., et al. 2001. Comparison of evidence of treatment effects in randomized and nonrandomized studies. *Journal of the American Medical Association* **286**: 821–30.

ISIS-2 (Second International Study of Infarct Survival) Collaborative Group. 1988. Randomised trial of intravenous streptokinase, oral aspirin, both, or neither among 17 187 cases of suspected acute myocardial infarction: ISIS-2. *Lancet* ii: 349–60.

Jadad, A.R., Cook, D.J., Jones, A., et al. 1998. Methodology and reports of systematic reviews and meta-analyses: a comparison of Cochrane reviews with articles published in paper-based journals. *Journal of the American Medical Association* **280**: 278–80.

Jadad, A.R., Moher, M., Browman, G.P., et al. 2000. Systematic reviews and meta-analyses on treatment of asthma: critical evaluation. *British Medical Journal* **320**: 537–40.

Jadad, A.R., Moore, R.A., Carroll, D., et al. 1996. Assessing the quality of reports of randomized clinical trials: is blinding necessary? *Controlled Clinical Trials* **17**: 1–12.

Johnson, P. 1983. What kind of expert should a system be? *Journal of Medicine and Philosophy* **8**: 77–97.

Jüni, P., Altman, D.G., and Egger, M. 2001. Assessing the quality of controlled clinical trials. *British Medical Journal* **323**: 42–6.

Jüni, P., Witschi, A., Bloch, R., and Egger, M. 1999. The hazards of scoring the quality of clinical trials for meta-analysis. *Journal of the American Medical Association* **282**: 1054–60.

Khoury, M.J., Burke, W., and Thomson, E.J., eds. 2000. *Genetics and Public Health in the 21st Century: Using Genetic Information to Improve Health and Prevent Disease.* Oxford: Oxford University Press.

King, H.C., and Sinha, A.A. 2001. Gene expression profile analysis by DNA microarrays: promise and pitfalls. *Journal of the American Medical Association* **286**: 2280–8.

King, M.C., Wieand, S., Hale, K., et al. 2001. Tamoxifen and breast cancer incidence among women with inherited mutations in BRCA1 and BRCA2: National Surgical Adjuvant Breast and Bowel Project (NSABP-P1) Breast Cancer Prevention Trial. *Journal of the American Medical Association* **286**: 2251–6.

Klausner, J.D., Wolf, W., Fischer-Ponce, L., Zolt, I., and Katz, M.H. 2000. Tracing a syphilis outbreak through cyberspace. *Journal of the American Medical Association* **284**: 447–9.

Knottnerus, J.A., and Dinant, G.J. 1997. Medicine based evidence, a prerequisite for evidence based medicine: future research methods must find ways of accommodating clinical reality, not ignoring it. *British Medical Journal* **315**: 1109–10.

Kohn, L.T, Corrigan, J.M., and Donaldson, M.S., eds. 2000. *To Err Is Human: Building a Safer Health System* (Committee on Quality of Health Care in America, Institute of Medicine) Washington, DC: National Academy Press.

Kolata, G. 2001. Study sets off debate over mammograms' value. *The New York Times*, National Edition, December 9: A1, A32.

Kuntz, K.M., Tsevat, J., Weinstein, M.C., and Goldman, L. 1999. Expert panel vs decision-analysis recommendations for postdischarge coronary angiography after myocardial infarction. *Journal of the American Medical Association* **282**: 2246–51.

Lamers, M.H., Kok, J.N, and Lebret, E. 1998. Combined neural network models for epidemiological data: modeling heterogeneity and reduction of input correlations. In *Proceedings of the Third International Conference on Artificial Neural Nets and Genetic Algorithms* (ICANNGA 97), ed. G.D. Smith, N.C. Steele, and R.F. Albrecht, pp. 147–51. New York: Springer-Verlag.

Langley, P., Simon, H.A., Bradshaw, G.L., and Zytkow, J.M. 1987. *Scientific Discovery: Computational Explorations of the Creative Processes.* Cambridge, Mass.: The MIT Press.

Lantos, J.D. 1997. *Do We Still Need Doctors?* New York: Routledge.

LaPorte, R.E., Marler, E., Akazawa, S., et al. 1995. The death of biomedical journals. *British Medical Journal* **310**: 1387–90.

Larkin, H. 1999. Not-in-practice guidelines. *American Medical News,* December 27, pp. 8, 10, 11.

Larkin, J., McDermott, J., Simon, D.P., and Simon, H.A.1980. Expert and novice performance in solving physics problems. *Science* **208**: 1335–42.

Lau, J., Antman, E.M., Jimenez-Silva, J., Kupelnick, B., Mosteller, F., and Chalmers, T.C. 1992. Cumulative meta-analysis of therapeutic trials for myocardial infarction. *New England Journal of Medicine* **327**: 248–54.

Laupacis, A., Sekar, N., and Stiell, I. 1997. Clinical prediction rules: a review and suggested modifications of methodological standards. *Journal of the American Medical Association* **277**: 488–94.

Lavrač, N. 1999. Selected techniques for data mining in medicine. *Artificial Intelligence in Medicine.* **16**: 3–23.

Leplin, J. ed. 1984. *Scientific Realism.* Berkeley, Calif.: University of California Press.

Light, R.J., and Pillemer, D.B. 1984. *Summing Up: The Science of Reviewing Research.* Cambridge, Mass.: Harvard University Press.

Linder, J.A., and Stafford, R.S. 2001. Antibiotic treatment of adults with sore throat by community primary care physicians: a national survey, 1989–1999. *Journal of the American Medical Association* **286**: 1181–6.

Logan, R.L., and Scott, P.J. 1996. Uncertainty on clinical practice: implications for quality and costs of health care. *Lancet* **347**: 595–8.

Lomas, J., Anderson, G.M., Dominick-Pierre, K., Vayda, E., Enkin, M.W., and Hannah, W.J. 1989. Do practice guidelines guide practice? *New England Journal of Medicine* **321**: 1306–11.

London, O. 1987. *Kill as Few Patients as Possible: And Fifty-Six Other Essays on How to Be the World's Best Doctor.* Berkeley, Calif.: Ten Speed Press.

Long, M.J. 2001. Clinical practice guidelines: when the tool becomes the rule. *Journal of Evaluation in Clinical Practice* **7**: 191–9.

Lord May. 2001. *Anniversary Address.* London: The Royal Society. Available at http://www.royalsoc.ac.uk/royalsoc/ann_2001.pdf.

Louis, P.C.A. 1834. *Essay on Clinical Instruction.*, transl. P. Martin, London: S. Highley. In *Medicine in Quotations: Views of Health and Disease Through the Ages*, ed. E.J. Huth and T.J. Murray. Philadelphia: American College of Physicians. Available at http://www.acponline.org/medquotes/index.html.

Lowe, M. 2000. Evidence-based medicine – the view from Fiji. *Lancet* **356**: 1105–7.

Maisonneuve, H., Codier, H., Durocher, A., and Matillon, Y. 1997. The French clinical guidelines and medical references programme: development of 48 guidelines for private practice over a period of 18 months. *Journal of Evaluation in Clinical Practice* **3**: 3–13.

Malakoff, D. 1999. Bayes offers a 'new' way to make sense of numbers. *Science* **286**: 1460–4.

Malin, B., and Sweeney, L. 2000. Determining the identifiability of DNA database entries. *Proceedings of the American Medical Informatics Association Annual Fall Symposium*, pp. 537–541.

Malterud, K. 2001. The art and science of clinical knowledge: evidence beyond measures and numbers. *Lancet* **358**: 397–400.

Mant, D. 1999. Can randomised trials inform clinical decisions about individual patients? *Lancet* **353**: 743–6.

Martin, B., and Richards, E. 1995. Scientific knowledge, controversy, and public decision-making. In *Handbook of Science and Technology Studies*, ed. S. Jasanoff et al., pp. 506–26, Newbury Park, Calif.: Russell Sage Foundation.

Matthews, J.R. 1999. Practice guidelines and tort reform: the legal system confronts the technocratic wish. *Journal of Health Politics, Policy and Law* **24**: 275–304.

McColl, A., Smith, H., White, P., and Field, J. 1998. General practitioners' perceptions of the route to evidence based medicine: a questionnaire survey. *British Medical Journal* **316**: 361–5.

McCray, A.T., and Ide, N.C. 2000. Design and implementation of a national clinical trials registry. *Journal of the American Medical Informatics Association* **7**: 313–23.

McDonald, C.J. 1996. Medical heuristics: the silent adjudicators of clinical practice. *Annals of Internal Medicine* **124**: 56–62.

McFarlane, M., Bull, S.S., and Rietmeijer, C.A. 2000. The Internet as a newly emerging risk environment for sexually transmitted diseases. *Journal of the American Medical Association* **284**: 443–6.

McGinn, T.G., Guyatt, G.H., Wyer, P.C., Naylor, C.D., Stiell, I.G., and Richardson, W.S. 2000. Users' guide to the medical literature. XXII: How to use articles about clinical decision rules. *Journal of the American Medical Association* **284**: 79–84.

McGuigan, S.M. 1995. The use of statistics in the *British Journal of Psychiatry*. *British Journal of Psychiatry* **167**: 683–8.

McNeil, B.J., Pauker, S.G., Sox, H.C., and Tversky, A. 1982. On the elicitation of preferences for alternative therapies. *New England Journal of Medicine* **306**: 1259–62.

McQuay, H.J., and Moore, R.A. 1997. Using numerical results from systematic reviews in clinical practice. *Annals of Internal Medicine* **126**: 712–20.

Mechanic, D. 2000. Managed care and the imperative for a new professional ethic. *Health Affairs* 19(5): 100–11.

Merz, J.F., Sankar, P., Taube, S.E., and Livolsi, V. 1997. Use of human tissues in research: clarifying clinician and researcher roles and information flows. *Journal of Investigative Medicine* 45: 252–7.

Mikulich, V.J., Liu, Y.-C.A., Steinfeldt, J., and Schriger, D.L. 2001. Implementation of clinical guidelines through an electronic medical record: physician usage, satisfaction and assessment. *International Journal of Medical Informatics* 63: 169–78.

Miller, R.A. 1990. Why the standard view is standard: people, not machines, understand patients' problems. *Journal of Medicine and Philosophy* 15: 581–91.

Miller, R., and Goodman, K.W. 1998. Ethical challenges in the use of decision-support software in clinical practice. In *Ethics, Computing and Medicine: Informatics and the Transformation of Health Care*, ed. K.W. Goodman, pp. 102–15. Cambridge and New York: Cambridge University Press.

Miller, R.A., Schaffner, K.F., and Meisel, A. 1985. Ethical and legal issues related to the use of computer programs in clinical medicine. *Annals of Internal Medicine* 102: 529–36.

Misselbrook, D., and Armstrong, D. 2001. Patients' responses to risk information about the benefits of treating hypertension. *British Journal of General Practice* 51: 276–9.

Mitchell, T.M. 1999. Machine learning and data mining. *Communications of the ACM* 42(11): 31–6.

Mjolsness, E., and DeCoste, D. 2001. Machine learning for science: state of the art and future prospects. *Science* 293: 2051–5.

Moher, D., Cook, D.J., Eastwood, S., Olkin, I., Rennie, D., and Stroup, D.F. 1999. Improving the quality of reports of meta-analyses of randomised controlled trials: the QUOROM statement. *Lancet* 354: 1896–900.

Moher, D., Jadad, A.R., Nichol, G., Penman, M., Tugwell, T., and Walsh, S. 1995. Assessing the quality of randomized controlled trials: an annotated bibliography of scales and checklists. *Controlled Clinical Trials* 16: 62–73.

Moher, D., Jadad, A.R., and Tugwell, P. 1996. Assessing the quality of randomized controlled trials: current issues and future directions. *International Journal of Technology Assessment in Health Care* 12: 195–208.

Moher, D., Jones, A., and Lepage, L. 2001 Use of the CONSORT statement and quality of reports of randomized trials: a comparative before-and-after evaluation. *Journal of the American Medical Association* 285: 1992–5.

Morreim, E.H. 2001a. From the clinics to the courts: the role evidence should play in litigating medical care. *Journal of Health Politics, Policy and Law* 26: 408–27.

Morreim, E.H. 2001b. Result-based compensation in health care: a good, but limited, idea. *Journal of Law, Medicine & Ethics* 29: 174–81.

Morris, A.H. 1998. Algorithm-based decision making. In *Principles and Practice of Intensive Care Monitoring*, ed. M.J. Tobin, pp. 1355–81. New York: McGraw-Hill.

Mosteller, F., and Tukey, J. 1977. *Data Analysis and Regression.* Boston: Addison Wesley.

Muir Gray, J.A. 1997. *Evidence-Based Healthcare.* Edinburgh: Churchill Livingstone.

Mulrow, C.D. 1987. The medical review article: state of the science. *Annals of Internal Medicine* **106**: 485–8.

Mulrow, C.D. 1995. Rational for systematic reviews. In *Systematic Reviews*, ed. I. Chalmers and D. Altman, pp. 1–8. London: BMJ Publishing Group.

Mulrow, C.D., Cook, D.J., and Davidoff, F. 1998. Systematic reviews: critical links in the great chain of evidence. In *Systematic Reviews: Synthesis of Best Evidence for Health Care Decisions*, ed. C. Mulrow and D. Cook, pp. 1–4. Philadelphia: American College of Physicians.

Mulrow, C.D., Langhorne, P., and Grimshaw, J. 1997. Integrating heterogeneous pieces of evidence in systematic reviews. *Annals of Internal Medicine* **127**: 989–95.

National Health Service. 2001. Centre for Evidence-Based Medicine. Available at http://cebm.jr2.ox.ac.uk/index.html.

National Institutes of Health Consensus Development Panel. 1997. National Institutes of Health Consensus Development Conference Statement: breast cancer screening for women ages 40–49, January 21–23, 1997. *Journal of the National Cancer Institute* **89**: 1015–26.

Nauwelaers, J. 2000. Eraritjaritjaka. *Lancet* **356**: 2169–70.

Nelson, J.L. 2000. In *Getting Doctors to Listen: Ethics and Outcomes Data in Context*, ed. P.J. Boyle, pp. 196–203. Hastings Center Studies in Ethics. Washington, DC: Georgetown University Press.

Newcombe, R.G. 1987. Towards a reduction in publication bias. *British Medical Journal* **295**: 656–9.

Newell, A., Shaw, J.C., and Simon, H.A. 1962. The processes of creative thinking. In *Contemporary Approaches to Creative Thinking*, ed. H.E. Gruber et al., pp. 63–119. New York: Atherton.

Noyes, H.D. 1865. Specialties in medicine. *Transactions of the American Ophthalmological Society* **2**: 59–74. Reprinted in *The Origins of Specialization in American Medicine*, ed. C.E. Rosenburg, pp. 3–18. New York: Garland (1989).

O'Donnell, M. 2000. Evidence-based illiteracy: time to rescue "the literature". *Lancet* **355**: 489–91.

Office of Technology Assessment. 1978. *Assessing the Efficacy and Safety of Medical Technologies.* (OTA-H-75). Washington, DC: Office of Technology Assessment.

Ohno-Machado, L., Gennari, J.H., Murphy, S.N., et al. 1998. The Guideline Interchange Format: a model for representing guidelines. *Journal of the American Medical Informatics Association* **5**: 357–72.

Olkin, I. 1990. History and goals. In *The Future of Meta-Analysis*, ed. K.W. Wachter and M.L. Straf, pp. 3–10. New York: Russell Sage Foundation.

Olkin, I. 1995. Meta-analysis: reconciling the results of independent studies. *Statistics in Medicine* **14**: 457–72.

Olsen, O., and Gøtzsche, P.C. 2001. Cochrane review on screening for breast cancer with mammography. *Lancet* **358**: 1340–2.

Olsen, O., Middleton, P., Ezzo, J., et al. 2001. Quality of Cochrane reviews: assessment of sample from 1998. *British Medical Journal* **323**: 829–32.

Osler, W. 1985. The influence of Louis on American medicine. In *The Collected Essays of Sir William Osler*, vol. III, ed. J.P. McGovern and C.G. Roland, pp. 113–34. Birmingham, Ala.: Classics of Medicine Library. Originally published in the *Johns Hopkins Hospital Bulletin*, Nos 77–78, August–September, 1897, pp. 189–210. (*Medicine in Quotations: Views of Health and Disease Through the Ages*, Cited in ed. E.J. Huth and T.J. Murray. Philadelphia: American College of Physicians. Available at http://www.acponline.org/medquotes/index.html).

Oxman, A. (in press) The Cochrane Collaboration: ten challenges, and one reason why they must be met. In *Systematic Reviews*, 2nd edn., ed. M. Egger, G.D. Smith, and D.G. Altman. London: BMJ Publications.

Oxman, A.D., and Guyatt, G.H. 1988. Guidelines for reading literature reviews. *Canadian Medical Association Journal* **138**: 697–703.

Padkin, A., Rowan, K., and Black, N. 2001. Using high quality clinical databases to complement the results of randomised controlled trials: the case of recombinant human activated protein C. *British Medical Journal* **323**: 923–6.

Patterson-Brown, S., Wyatt, J.C., and Fisk, N.M. 1993. Are clinicians interested in up to date reviews of effective care? *British Medical Journal* **307**: 1464.

Pearson, K. 1904. Report on certain enteric fever inoculation statistics. *British Medical Journal* **2**: 1243–6.

Pearson, K. 1905. *National Life From the Standpoint of Science*. London: University Press.

Peirce, C.S. 1958. *Collected Papers of Charles Sanders Peirce*, Vol. VII., ed. A.W. Burks. Cambridge, Mass.: Harvard University Press.

Petitti, D.B. 2000. *Meta-analysis, Decision Analysis, and Cost-effectiveness Analysis: Methods for Quantitative Synthesis in Medicine*, 2nd edn. Oxford: Oxford University Press.

Peto, R., Collins, R., and Gray, R. 1995. Large-scale randomized evidence: large, simple trials and overviews of trials. *Journal of Clinical Epidemiology* **48**: 23–40.

Petticrew, M. 2001. Systematic reviews from astronomy to zoology: myths and misconceptions. *British Medical Journal* **322**: 98–101.

Petticrew, M., Song, F., Wilson, P., and Wright, K. 1999. Quality-assessed reviews of health care interventions and the Database of Abstracts of Reviews of Effectiveness (DARE). *International Journal of Technology Assessment in Health Care* **15**: 671–8.

Pfeifer, M.P., and Snodgrass, G.L. 1990. The continued use of retracted, invalid scientific literature. *Journal of the American Medical Association* **263**: 1420–3.

Phillips, B., Ball, C., Sackett, D., Badenoch, D., Straus, S., and Haynes, B. 2001. Levels of evidence and grades of recommendations. Oxford Centre for Evidence-based Medicine. Available at http://cebm.jr2.ox.ac.uk/docs/levels.html.

Phillips, K.A., Veenstra, D.L., Oren, E., Lee, J.K., and Sadee, W. 2001. Potential role of pharmacogenomics in reducing adverse drug reactions: a systematic review. *Journal of the American Medical Association* **286**: 2270–9.

Pillemer, D.B., and Light, R.L. 1980. Synthesizing outcomes: how to use research evidence from many studies. *Harvard Educational Review* **50**: 176–95.

Pitkin, R.M., Branagan, M.A., and Burmeister, L.F. 1999. Accuracy of data in abstracts of published research articles. *Journal of the American Medical Association* **281**: 1110–11.

Plsek, P.E., and Greenhalgh, T. 2001. The challenge of complexity in health care. *British Medical Journal* **323**: 625–8.

Pocock, S.J., and Elbourne, D.R. 2000. Randomized trials or observational tribulations? *New England Journal of Medicine* **342**: 1907–9.

Popkin, R.H. 1967. Skepticism. In *The Encyclopedia of Philosophy*, Vol. 7, ed. P. Edwards, pp. 449–61. New York: Macmillan.

Porter, A.M.W. 1999. Misuse of correlation and regression in three medical journals. *Journal of the Royal College of Medicine* **92**: 123–8.

Porter, R. 1992. The rise of medical journalism in Britain to 1800. In *Medical Journals and Medical Knowledge: Historical Essays*, ed. W.F. Bynum, S. Lock and R. Porter, pp. 6–28. London and New York: Routledge.

Porter, R. 1996. Medical science. In *The Cambridge Illustrated History of Medicine*, ed. R. Porter, pp. 154–201. Cambridge: Cambridge University Press.

President's Advisory Commission on Consumer Protection and Quality in the Health Care Industry. 1998. *Quality First: Better Health Care for All Americans*. Washington, D.C.: U.S. Government Printing Office.

Putnam, H. 1970. Is semantics possible? *Metaphilosophy* **1**: 187–201.

Putnam, H. 1975. *Mathematics, Matter and Method: Philosophical Papers*, Vol. 1. Cambridge: Cambridge University Press.

Quine, W.V.O. 1953. *From a Logical Point of View*. Cambridge, Mass.: Harvard University Press.

Redelmeier, D.A., and Tversky, A. 1990. Discrepancy between medical decisions for individual patients and for groups. *New England Journal of Medicine* **322**: 1162–4.

Reid, M.C., Lane, D.A., and Feinstein, A.R. 1998. Academic calculations versus clinical judgments: practicing physicians' use of quantitative measures of test accuracy. *American Journal of Medicine* **104**: 374–80.

Richards, G., Rayward-Smith, V.J., Sönksen, P.H., Carey, S., and Weng, C. 2001. Data mining for indicators of early mortality in a database of clinical records. *Artificial Intelligence in Medicine* **22**: 215–31.

Rodwin, M.A. 2001. The politics of evidence-based medicine. *Journal of Health Politics, Policy and Law* **26**: 439–46.

Rosenbaum, S., Frankford, D.M., Moore, B., and Borzi, P. 1999. Who should determine when health care is medically necessary? *New England Journal of Medicine* **340**: 229–32.

Rosenberg, C.E., ed. 1989. *The Origins of Specialization in American Medicine: An Anthology of Sources.* New York and London: Garland Publishing.

Rosendaal, F.R. 1994. The emergence of a new species: the professional meta-analyst. *Journal of Clinical Epidemiology* 47: 1325–6.

Rosoff, A.J. 1995. The role of clinical practice guidelines in health care reform. *Health Matrix: Journal of Law-Medicine* 5: 369–96.

Rosoff, A.J. 2001. Evidence-based medicine and the law: the courts confront clinical practice guidelines. *Journal of Health Politics, Policy and Law* 26: 327–68.

Ross, J.W. 2000. Practice guidelines: texts in search of authority. In *Getting Doctors to Listen: Ethics and Outcomes Data in Context*, ed. P.J. Boyle, pp. 41–70. Hastings Center Studies in Ethics. Washington, DC: Georgetown University Press.

Ryan, T.J., Antman, E.M., Brooks, N.H., et al. 1999 update: ACC/AHA guidelines for the management of patients with acute myocardial infarction: executive summary and recommendations: a report of the American College of Cardiology/American Heart Association Task Force on Practice Guidelines (Committee on Management of Acute Myocardial Infarction). *Circulation* 100: 1016–30.

Sackett, D.L., Haynes, R.B., Guyatt, G.H., and Tugwell, P. 1991. *Clinical Epidemiology: A Basic Science for Clinical Medicine.* Boston: Little, Brown.

Sackett, D.L., Rosenberg, W.M.C., Muir Gray, J.A., Haynes, R.B., and Richardson, W.S. 1996. Evidence-based medicine: what it is and what it isn't. *British Medical Journal* 312: 71–2.

Sackett, D.L., Straus, S.E., Richardson, W.S., Rosenberg, W., and Haynes, R.B. 2000. *Evidence-Based Medicine: How to Practice and Teach EBM*, 2nd edn. Edinburgh: Churchill Livingstone.

Sacks, H.S., Berrier, J., Reitman, D., Ancona-Berk, V.A., and Chalmers, T.C. 1987. Meta-analyses of randomized controlled trials. *New England Journal of Medicine* 316: 450–5.

Sacks, H.S., Berrier, J. , Reitman, D., Pagano, D., and Chalmers, T.C. 1992. Meta-analyses of randomized control trials: an update of the quality and methodology. In *Medical Uses of Statistics*, 2nd edn, ed. J.C. Bailar III and F. Mosteller, pp. 427–42. Boston: NEJM Books.

Salmon, W.C. 1984. *Scientific Explanation and the Causal Structure of the World.* Princeton: Princeton University Press.

Salmon, W.C. 1998. Scientific explanation: causation and unification. In *Causality and Explanation*, ed. W.C. Salmon, pp. 68–78. New York and Oxford: Oxford University Press, Originally published in *Critica* (1990) 22(66): 3–21.

Sanders, G.D., Nease, R.F., and Owens, D.K. 2000. Design and pilot evaluation of a system to develop computer-based site-specific practice guidelines from decision models. *Medical Decision Making* 20: 145–59.

Sargent, D.J., Goldberg, R.M., Jacobson, S.D., et al. 2001. A pooled analysis of adjuvant chemotherapy for resected colon cancer in elderly patients. *New England Journal of Medicine* 345: 1091–7.

Schulze-Kremer, S. 1999. Discovery in the Human Genome Project. *Communications of the ACM* 42(11): 62–4.

Shaneyfelt, T.M., Mayo-Smith, M.F., and Rothwangl, J. 1999. Are guidelines following guidelines? The methodological quality of clinical practice guidelines in the peer-reviewed medical literature. *Journal of the American Medical Association* 281: 1900–5.

Shapiro, S. 1994. Meta-analysis/shmeta-analysis. *American Journal of Epidemiology* 140: 771–8.

Sharpe, V.A., and Faden, A.I. 1998. *Medical Harm: Historical, Conceptual, and Ethical Dimensions of Iatrogenic Illness.* Cambridge: Cambridge University Press.

Shaywitz, D.A., and Ausiello, D.A. 2001. The necessary risks of medical research. *The New York Times,* National Edition, July 29, section 4, p. 4.

Shekelle, P.G., Woolf, S.H., Eccles, M., and Grimshaw, J. 1999. Developing guidelines. *British Medical Journal* 318: 593–6.

Siang, S. 2000. Researching ethically with human subjects in cyberspace. *Professional Ethics Report* 12(4): 1, 7–8 (Newsletter of the Scientific Freedom, Responsibility and Law Program, American Association for the Advancement of Science, Washington, DC).

Silagy, C.A., Stead, L.F., and Lancaster, T. 2001. Use of systematic reviews in clinical practice guidelines: case study of smoking cessation. *British Medical Journal* 323: 833–6.

Simes, R.J. 1986. Publication bias: the case for an international registry of clinical trials. *Journal of Clinical Oncology* 4: 1529–41.

Simon, H.A. 1997a. *Models of Bounded Rationality,* Vol. 3. Cambridge, Mass.: The MIT Press.

Simon, H.A. 1997b. *Administrative Behavior,* 4th edn. New York: The Free Press.

Simon, H.A. 1999. *The Sciences of the Artificial,* 3rd edn. Cambridge, Mass.: The MIT Press.

Singer, P., McKie, J., Kuhse, H., and Richardson, J. 1995. Double jeopardy and the QALYs in health care allocation. *Journal of Medical Ethics* 21: 144–50.

Smalheiser, N.R., and Swanson, D.R. 1998. Using ARROWSMITH: a computer-assisted approach to formulating and assessing scientific hypotheses. *Computer Methods and Programs in Biomedicine* 57: 149–53.

Smith, R. 1992. The ethics of ignorance. *Journal of Medical Ethics* 18: 117–18, 134.

Smith, R., and Horton, R. 1999. Time to register randomised trials. *British Medical Journal* 319: 865–6 (version of Horton and Smith 1999).

Sox, H.C., and Woloshin, S. 2000. How many deaths are due to medical error? Getting the number right. *Effective Clinical Practice* 6: 277–83.

Spinler, S.A., Hilleman, D.E., Cheng, J.W.M., et al. 2001. New recommendations from the 1999 American College of Cardiology/American Heart Association acute myocardial infarction guidelines. *Annals of Pharmacotherapy* 35: 589–617.

Stein, B., and Fuster, V. 1992. Clinical pharmacology of platelet inhibitors. In *Thrombosis in Cardiovascular Disorders,* ed. V. Fuster and M. Verstraete, pp. 99–119. Philadelphia: WB Saunders.

Steinberg, K.K., Smith, S.J., Stroup, D.F., et al. 1997. Comparison of effect estimates from a meta-analysis of summary data from published studies and from a meta-analysis using individual patient data for ovarian cancer studies. *American Journal of Epidemiology* 145: 917–25.

Sterne, J.A.C., Egger, M., and Smith, G.D. 2001. Systematic reviews in health care: investigating and dealing with publication and other biases in meta-analysis. *British Medical Journal* 323: 101–5.

Stool, S.E., Berg, A.O., and Berman, S. 1994. *Otitis media with effusion in young children.* Clinical practice guideline, number 12. Rockville, MD: Agency for Health Care Policy and Research.

Stoto, M.A. 2000. Research synthesis for public health policy: experience of the Institute of Medicine. In *Meta-Analysis in Medicine and Health Policy*, ed. D.K. Stangl and D.A. Berry, pp. 321–57. New York: Marcel Dekker.

Stross, J.K. 1999. Guidelines have their limits. *Annals of Internal Medicine* 131: 304–5.

Susser, M., and Yankauer, A. 1993. Prior, duplicate, repetitive, fragmented, and redundant publication and editorial decisions. *American Journal of Public Health* 83: 792–3.

Sutton, A.J., Duval, S.J., Tweedie, R.L., Abrams, K.R., and Jones, D.R. 2000. Empirical assessment of effect of publication bias on meta-analyses. *British Medical Journal* 320: 1574–7.

Sweeney, L.A. 1997. Guaranteeing anonymity when sharing medical data: the Datafly System. *Proceedings of American Medical Informatics Association Annual Fall Symposium*, pp. 51–5.

Szolovits, P. 1995. Uncertainty and decisions in medical informatics. *Methods of Information in Medicine* 34: 111–21.

Takata, G.S., Chan, L.S., and Shekelle, P. 2001. Evidence assessment of management of acute otitis media: I. The role of antibiotics in treatment of uncomplicated acute otitis media. *Pediatrics* 108: 239–47.

Tanenbaum, S.J. 1993. What physicians know. *New England Journal of Medicine* 329: 1268–71.

Tanenbaum, S. J. 1994. Knowing and acting in medical practice: the epistemological politics of outcomes research. *Journal of Health Politics, Policy and Law* 19: 27–44.

Taylor, L. 1982. Trial and error: the very essence of life. *The Times*, London, July 26, p. 7.

Terenziani, P., Molino, G., and Torchio, M. 2001. A modular approach for representing and executing clinical guidelines. *Artificial Intelligence in Medicine* 23: 249–76.

Thompson, S.G. 1994. Why sources of heterogeneity in meta-analysis should be investigated. *British Medical Journal* 309: 1351–5.

Thomson, R., Parkin, D., Eccles, M., Sudlow, M., and Robinson, A. 2000. Decision analysis and guidelines for anticoagulant therapy to prevent stroke in patients with atrial fibrillation. *Lancet* 355: 956–62.

Tiles, J.E. 1984. Technē and moral expertise. *Philosophy* 59: 49–66.

Tramèr, M.R., Moore, R.A., Reynolds, D.J.M., and McQuay, H.J. 1997. A quantitative systematic review of ondansetron in treatment of established postoperative nausea and vomiting. *British Medical Journal* **314**: 1088–92.

TROUT Review Group. 2001. How do the outcomes of patients treated within randomised control trials compare with those of similar patients treated outside these trials? Available at http://hiru.mcmaster.ca/ebm/trout/

Tunis, S.R., Hayward, R.S.A., Wilson, M.C., Rubin, H.R., Bass, E.B., and Johnston, M. 1994. Internists' attitudes about clinical practice guidelines. *Annals of Internal Medicine* **120**: 956–63.

Tuttle, J. 1995. Sir Humphrey Davy (1778–1829). The Royal Institution of Great Britain website. Available at http://www.ri.ac.uk/History/.

Tversky, A., and Kahneman, D. 1974. Judgment under uncertainty: heuristics and biases. *Science* **185**: 1124–31.

Ubel, P.A., and Lowenstein, G. 1997. The role of decision analysis in informed consent: Choosing between intuition and systematicity. *Social Science and Medicine* **44**: 647–56.

Ubel, P.A., Dekay, M.L., Baron, J., and Asch, D.A. 1996. Cost-effectiveness analysis in a setting of budget constraints: is it equitable? *New England Journal of Medicine* **334**: 1174–7.

University of Minnesota. 2001. Florence Nightingale (1820–1910). Available at 2001http://www.mrs.umn.edu/~sungurea/introstat/history/w98/Nightingale.html

Vandenbroucke, J.P. 1998. Medical journals and the shaping of medical knowledge. *Lancet* **352**: 2001–6.

Villar, J., Mackey, M.E., Carroli, G., and Donner, A. 2001. Meta-analyses in systematic reviews of randomized controlled trials in perinatal medicine: comparison of fixed and random effects models. *Statistics in Medicine* **20**: 3635–47.

Von Staden, H. 1996. "In a pure and holy way:" Personal and professional conduct in the Hippocratic Oath. *Journal of the History of Medicine and Allied Sciences* **51**: 406–8.

Wachter, K.W. 1988. Disturbed by meta-analysis? *Science* **241**: 1407–8.

Wachter, K.W., and Straf, M.L., eds. 1990. *The Future of Meta-Analysis*. New York: Russell Sage Foundation.

Wagner, M.M., Tsui, F.-C., Espino, J.U., et al. 2001. The emerging science of very early detection of disease outbreaks. *Journal of Public Health Management and Practice* **7**(6): 50–8.

Warren, K.S., and Mosteller, F., eds. 1993. *Doing More Good than Harm: The Evaluation of Health Care Interventions*. Annals of the New York Academy of Sciences, Vol. 703. New York: New York Academy of Sciences.

Weatherall, M. 1996. Drug treatment and the rise in pharmacology. In *The Cambridge Illustrated History of Medicine*, ed. R. Porter, pp. 246–77. Cambridge: Cambridge University Press.

Weinberger, M., and Hui, S.L. eds. 1997. Measuring quality, outcomes, and cost of care using large databases: the sixth Regenstrief conference. *Annals of Internal Medicine* **127**(8.2): 666–774.

Weingarten, S. 1997. Practice guidelines and prediction rules should be subject to careful clinical testing. *Journal of the American Medical Association* 277: 1977–8.

Welch, G.E., and Gabbe, S.G. 1996. Review of statistics usage in the *American Journal of Obstetrics and Gynecology*. *American Journal of Obstetrics and Gynecology* 175: 1138–41.

Wennberg, J.E. 1984. Dealing with medical practice variation: a proposal for action. *Health Affairs* 3(2): 6–32.

Wennberg, J., and Gittelsohn, A. 1973. Small area variations in health care delivery. *Science* 182: 1102–8.

Wennberg, J., and Gittelsohn, A. 1982. Variations in medical care among small areas. *Scientific American* 246(4): 120–34.

Wilks, Y., Fass, D., Guo, C.M., McDonald, J., Plate, T., and Slator, B. 1990. A tractable machine dictionary as a basis for computational semantics. *Machine Translation* 5: 99–154.

Wilson, T., and Holt, T. 2001. Complexity and clinical care. *British Medical Journal* 323: 685–8.

Wilson, M.C., Hayward, R.S.A., Tunis, S.R., Bass, E.B., and Guyatt, G., for the Evidence-Based Medicine Working Group. 1995. Users' guides to the medical literature. VIII: how to use clinical practice guidelines; B: what are the recommendations and will they help you in caring for your patients? *Journal of the American Medical Association* 274: 1630–2.

Wittgenstein, L. 1968. *Philosophical Investigations,* 3rd edn, transl. G.E.M. Anscombe. Oxford: Blackwell.

Woolf, S.H. 1993. Practice guidelines: a new reality in medicine. *Archives of Internal Medicine* 153: 2646–55.

Woolf, S.H. 1998. Do clinical practice guidelines define good medical care? The need for good science and the disclosure of uncertainty when defining "best practices." *Chest* 113: 166S-71S.

Woolf, S.H. 1999. The need for perspective in evidence-based medicine. *Journal of the American Medical Association* 282: 2358–65.

Woolf, S.H., and Lawrence, R.S. 1997. Preserving scientific debate and patient choice: lessons from the Consensus Panel on mammography screening. *Journal of the American Medical Association* 278: 2105–8.

Woolf, S.H., Grol, R., Hutchinson, A., Eccles, M., and Grimshaw, J. 1999. Potential benefits, limitations, and harms of clinical guidelines. *British Medical Journal* 318: 527–30.

Yoshioka, A. 1998. Use of randomisation in the Medical Research Council's clinical trial of streptomycin in pulmonary tuberculosis in the 1940s. *British Medical Journal* 317: 1220–3.

Ziman, J.M. 1986. Getting to know everything about nothing. In *Progress in Science and Its Social Conditions*, ed. T. Ganelius, pp. 93–109. Oxford: Pergamon Press.

Index